■ ERRATA ■

BENZODIAZEPINES AND GHB
Detection and Pharmacology

Edited by
Salvatore J. Salamone

Chapter 2, Immunoassay of Benzodiazepines

PAGE 20: The image above the legend for Fig. 1 is actually Fig. 3 and should appear above the legend for Fig. 3 on page 30.

PAGE 20: In the legend for Fig. 1, the following key to symbols should be inserted: "(●) lorazepam-glucuronide; (■) oxazepam-glucuronide; (▲) temazepam-glucuronide."

PAGE 21: The image above the legend for Fig. 2 is actually Fig. 1 and should appear above the legend for Fig. 1 on page 20.

PAGE 21: In the legend for Fig. 2, the following key to symbols should be inserted: "(●) lorazepam-glucuronide; (■) oxazepam-glucuronide; (▲) temazepam-glucuronide."

PAGE 21: At the bottom of the page, substitute the following for the last paragraph and equation:

"The following generalized equation can be used to calculate the quantity of glucuronidated benzodiazepine hydrolyzed in different applications of the automated hydrolysis procedure when using international units (U) of enzyme:

$$1/A \times B \times 5 \times 10^8 = \text{ng/mL of BG hydrolyzed per U}"$$

PAGE 26: Substitute the following for the final paragraph:

"The SBENZ assay also has a serum application with a 3 ng/mL LOD. This LOD has been shown to be very effective in detecting low levels of low-dose benzodiazepines *(17,24)*. In one study, single doses of flunitrazepam were detected over a 72-h period in serum and the clinical sensitivity was shown to be similar to GC/MS *(24)*. In addition, a second calibration is not required when the matrix is changed from urine to serum or saliva *(17)*."

PAGE 27: Substitute the following for the first line of the table body: "Concentration <300 ng/mL"

PAGE 29: In the last paragraph, in the fourth sentence, substitute "immunoassay itself" for "benzodiazepine assay." Also, substitute the reference citation number *10* for *4* in the last two sentences.

PAGE 30: The image above the legend for Fig. 3 is actually Fig. 2 and should appear above the legend for Fig. 2 on page 21.

Benzodiazepines and GHB

FORENSIC SCIENCE AND MEDICINE

Steven B. Karch, MD, SERIES EDITOR

BUPRENORPHINE THERAPY OF OPIATE ADDICTION,
  edited by *PASCAL KINTZ AND PIERRE MARQUET, 2002*
ON-SITE DRUG TESTING,
  edited by *AMANDA J. JENKINS AND BRUCE A. GOLDBERGER, 2001*
BENZODIAZEPINES AND GHB: *DETECTION AND PHARMACOLOGY,*
  edited by *Salvatore J. Salamone, 2001*
TOXICOLOGY AND CLINICAL PHARMACOLOGY OF HERBAL PRODUCTS,
  edited by *Melanie Johns Cupp, 2000*
CRIMINAL POISONING: *INVESTIGATIONAL GUIDE FOR LAW ENFORCEMENT, TOXICOLOGISTS, FORENSIC SCIENTISTS, AND ATTORNEYS,*
  by *John H. Trestrail, III, 2000*
A PHYSICIAN'S GUIDE TO CLINICAL FORENSIC MEDICINE,
  edited by *Margaret M. Stark, 2000*

BENZODIAZEPINES AND GHB

Detection and Pharmacology

Edited by

Salvatore J. Salamone, PhD

*Roche Diagnostics Corp.
Indianapolis, IN*

Humana Press 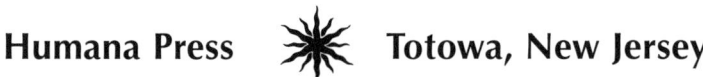 Totowa, New Jersey

To my children Katherine, Norah, and Hannah

© 2001 Humana Press Inc.
999 Riverview Drive, Suite 208
Totowa, New Jersey 07512

www.humanapress.com

All rights reserved. No part of this book may be reproduced, stored in a retrieval system, or transmitted in any form or by any means, electronic, mechanical, photocopying, microfilming, recording, or otherwise without written permission from the Publisher.

The content and opinions expressed in this book are the sole work of the authors and editors, who have warranted due diligence in the creation and issuance of their work. The publisher, editors, and authors are not responsible for errors or omissions or for any consequences arising from the information or opinions presented in this book and make no warranty, express or implied, with respect to its contents.

This publication is printed on acid-free paper. ∞
ANSI Z39.48-1984 (American Standards Institute) Permanence of Paper for Printed Library Materials.

Cover design by Patricia F. Cleary.

For additional copies, pricing for bulk purchases, and/or information about other Humana titles, contact Humana at the above address or at any of the following numbers: Tel: 973-256-1699; Fax: 973-256-8341; E-mail: humana@humanapr.com, or visit our Website at www.humanapress.com

Photocopy Authorization Policy:

Authorization to photocopy items for internal or personal use, or the internal or personal use of specific clients, is granted by Humana Press Inc., provided that the base fee of US $10.00 per copy, plus US $00.25 per page, is paid directly to the Copyright Clearance Center at 222 Rosewood Drive, Danvers, MA 01923. For those organizations that have been granted a photocopy license from the CCC, a separate system of payment has been arranged and is acceptable to Humana Press Inc. The fee code for users of the Transactional Reporting Service is: [0-89603-981-1/01 $10.00 + $00.25].

Printed in the United States of America. 10 9 8 7 6 5 4 3 2 1

Library of Congress Cataloging in Publication Data

Benzodiazepines and GHB: detection and pharmacology
  p. ; cm. -- (Forensic science and medicine)
  Includes bibliographical references and index.
  ISBN 0-89603-981-1 (alk. paper)
  1. Benzodiazepines--Analysis. 2. Gamma-hydroxybutyrate--Analysis. 3. Forensic pharmacology. I. Salamone, Salvatore J. II. Series.
  [DNLM: 1. Body Fluids--chemistry. 2. Forensic Medicine--methods. 3. Benzodiazepines--isolation & purification. 4. Benzodiazepines--metabolism. 5. Benzodiazepines--pharmacology. 6. Hair--chemistry. 7. Hydroxybutyrates--isolation & purification. 8. Hydroxybutyrates--metabolism. 9. Hydroxybutyrates--pharmacology. W 750 D4799 2001]
  RA1242.B43 D48 2001
  614'.1--dc21

2001024305

Preface

Since the first benzodiazepines were introduced to the market in 1960, there has been an evolution of these drugs toward lower dosage, shorter action, and faster clearance. As a consequence, this new generation of benzodiazepines eluded detection in many laboratories. Benzodiazepines can be abused in several different ways. These drugs are often given in conjunction with alcohol to enhance the desired effect, thus requiring lower doses. This situation has created added challenges to the toxicologist. Use of normal screening and confirmation methods may not detect the lower levels of these drugs, and in some cases the laboratory may not have capability in the methodologies to detect a particular drug.

Another recent challenge for the toxicologist is the detection of γ-hydroxybutyric acid (GHB). The use of this drug is widespread and it is easily obtained or prepared in clandestine laboratories. Similar to the low-dosed benzodiazepines (LDBs) the effect is also potentiated by alcohol. Its detection is difficult owing to the rapid clearance and the low concentrations that appear in urine or serum. Detection methods for GHB are not common, but laboratories are now developing new methods as its popularity is highlighted.

The purpose of *Benzodiazepines and GHB: Detection and Pharmacology* is to provide some background on the pharmacology and metabolism of LDB and GHB and to help the toxicologist develop methodologies that will enable better detection of these drugs in various body fluids, as well as in hair. The first chapter provides background on the LDBs by dealing with the pharmacology and metabolism of these drugs. Chapter 2 deals with immunoassay detection of LDBs, reviewing the current state of testing and providing methodologies that will increase the sensitivity of immunoassay reagents. Chapters 3 and 4 focus on methods for the detection of Rohypnol® and other LDBs by mass spectrometry. Chapter 5 addresses the detection of benzodiazepines in hair. Chapter 6 addresses the pharmacology and detection of GHB, and finally

Chapter 7 presents a case study examining the prevalence of drugs used in cases of alleged sexual assault.

Benzodiazepines and GHB: Detection and Pharmacology would not have been possible without the cooperation of all the authors. I wish to thank each of them for their efforts. I would like to thank Dr. Stephen Karch and Humana Press for the opportunity to be involved with such an endeavor.

Salvatore J. Salamone, PhD

Contents

Preface v

Contributors xi

CHAPTER 1

Pharmacology of Flunitrazepam and Other Benzodiazepines

Rudolf Brenneisen and Lionel Raymond 1

    1. Introduction 1
    2. Chemistry 2
    3. Pharmacokinetics 4
        3.1. Absorption, Distribution, and Plasma Levels 4
        3.2. Half-Life vs Duration of Action 7
        3.3. Metabolism and Excretion 7
    4. Pharmacodynamics 8
        4.1. Sites of Action 8
        4.2. Acute Effect 10
        4.3. Chronic Administration and Abuse Liability 11
        4.4. Pharmacokinetics vs Pharmacodynamics 12
        4.5. Rohypnol®: The Debate 13
    References 14

CHAPTER 2

Immunoassay Detection of Benzodiazepines

Tamara N. St. Claire and Salvatore J. Salamone 17

1. Introduction 17
2. Optimal Enzyme Activity 19
    2.1. Conditions 19
    2.2. Activity 20
3. Cutoff 22
4. Immunoassays 22
5. Methods 28
    5.1. Manual β-Glucuronidase Treatment 28
    5.2. Automated β-Glucuronidase Treatment 28
        5.2.1. Online with the Hitachi 717 28
        5.2.2. Online with the COBAS INTEGRA 700 29
        5.2.3. A General Scheme 29
6. Conclusion 29
References 30

CHAPTER 3

Analysis of Flunitrazepam and Its Metabolites in Biological Specimens

Mahmoud A. ElSohly and Shixia Feng 33

1. Introduction 33
2. Methods of Analysis 35
    2.1. Screening Methods 35
    2.2. HPLC Analysis 37
        2.2.1. Internal Standards 37
        2.2.2. Extraction 38
        2.2.3. HPLC Conditions 41
        2.2.4. Detection 42
    2.3. GC/MS Methods 43
3. Conclusion 48
References 49

Chapter 4
Analysis of Selected Low-Dose Benzodiazepines by Mass Spectrometry

Dennis J. Crouch and Matthew H. Slawson 53

    1. Introduction 53
    2. Alprazolam 55
        2.1. Background 55
        2.2. Method 1 57
            2.2.1. Extraction 57
            2.2.2. GC/MS Conditions 58
            2.2.3. Method Performance 58
        2.3. Method 2 59
            2.3.1. Extraction 60
            2.3.2. HPLC/MS/MS Conditions 60
            2.3.3. Method Performance 60
    3. Midazolam 63
        3.1. Background 63
        3.2. Method 1 63
            3.2.1. Extraction 63
            3.2.2. GC/MS Conditions 64
            3.2.3. Method Performance 64
        3.3. Method 2 64
            3.3.1. Extraction 64
            3.3.2. HPLC/MS Conditions 64
            3.3.3. Method Performance 65
        3.4. Method 3 65
            3.4.1. Extraction 65
            3.4.2. HPLC/MS Conditions 65
            3.4.3. Method Performance 65
        3.5. Additional Techniques 65
    4. Lorazepam 66
        4.1. Background 66
        4.2. Method 66
            4.2.1. Extraction 66
            4.2.2. GC/MS Conditions 67
            4.2.3. Method Performance 67
        4.3. Additional Techniques 67
    5. Triazolam 68
        5.1. Background 68
        5.2. Method 1 70
            5.2.1. Extraction 70
            5.2.2. GC/MS Conditions 70
            5.2.3. Method Performance 70
        5.3. Method 2 71
            5.3.1. Extraction 71
            5.3.2. GC/MS Conditions 71
            5.3.3. Method Performance 71
    References 71

Chapter 5

Identification of Benzodiazepines in Human Hair: *A Review*

Vincent Cirimele and Pascal Kintz 77

1. Introduction 77
2. Biology of Hair 78
   2.1. Hair Growth 78
   2.2. Types of Hair 79
   2.3. Mechanisms of Drug Incorporation into Hair 79
   2.4. Effects of Cosmetic Treatments 80
3. Specimen Collection 81
4. Decontamination Procedures 81
5. Extraction 81
6. Detection 84
7. Detection of Flunitrazepam and 7-Amino-Flunitrazepam 90
8. Conclusions 92
References 92

Chapter 6

γ-Hydroxybutyric Acid and Its Analogs, γ-Butyrolactone and 1,4-Butanediol

Laureen J. Marinetti 95

1. History and Pharmacology of GHB 95
2. History of Illicit Use of GHB 98
3. Clinical Use of GHB in Humans 101
4. History of Illicit Use of GBL and 1,4BD 102
5. Metabolism of GHB, GBL, and 1,4BD 104
6. Distribution and Pharmacokinetics of GHB, GBL, and 1,4BD 108
7. GHB Interpretation Issues and Postmortem Production 110
8. Analysis for GHB, GBL, and 1,4BD 115
References 119

Chapter 7

Analysis of Urine Samples in Cases of Alleged Sexual Assault: *Case History*

Mahmoud A. ElSohly, Luen F. Lee, Lynn B. Holzhauer, and Salvatore J. Salamone 127

1. Introduction 127
2. Receipt of Specimens for Analysis 128
3. Testing Protocol 129
4. Results and Discussion 131
5. Conclusions 142
References 143

Index *145*

Contributors

RUDOLF BRENNEISEN • Department of Clinical Research, University of Bern, Bern, Switzerland

VINCENT CIRIMELE • Institute of Legal Medicine, University of Strasbourg, Strasbourg, France

DENNIS J. CROUCH • Center for Human Toxicology, University of Utah, Salt Lake City, UT

MAHMOUD A. ELSOHLY • ElSohly Laboratories, Oxford, MS

SHIXIA FENG • ElSohly Laboratories, Oxford, MS

LYNN B. HOLZHAUER • Statistics and Data Management, Roche Pharmaceuticals, Nutley, NJ

PASCAL KINTZ • Institute of Legal Medicine, University of Strasbourg, Strasbourg, France

LUEN F. LEE • Statistics and Data Management, Roche Pharmaceuticals, Nutley, NJ

LAUREEN J. MARINETTI • College of Pharmacy and Allied Health Professions, Wayne State University; Wayne County Medical Examiner's Office, Detroit, MI

LIONEL RAYMOND • Forensic Toxicology Laboratory, University of Miami, Miami, FL

SALVATORE J. SALAMONE • Research and Development, Roche Diagnostics Corp., Indianapolis, IN

MATTHEW H. SLAWSON • Center for Human Toxicology, University of Utah, Salt Lake City, UT

TAMARA N. ST. CLAIRE • Research and Development, Roche Diagnostics Corp., Indianapolis, IN

Chapter 1

Pharmacology of Flunitrazepam and Other Benzodiazepines

Rudolf Brenneisen and Lionel Raymond

1. Introduction

Benzodiazepines, therapeutically used as tranquilizers, hypnotics, anticonvulsants, and centrally acting muscle relaxants, rank among the most frequently prescribed drugs *(1)*. Since Sternbach's synthesis *(2)* in 1955 of the first benzodiazepine by unexpected ring extension of a quinazoline-3-*N*-oxide derivative, a number of structurally similar compounds have been marketed by drug companies. Chlordiazepoxide (Librium®) was the first medical benzodiazepine, introduced in 1960, followed in 1963 by diazepam (Valium®) and in 1965 by oxazepam (Serax®) *(2)*. More than 50 of these drugs are presently marketed for clinical use throughout the world; 35 are subject to international control under the 1971 Convention on Psychotropic Substances. From International Narcotic Control Board (INCB) statistics, the most significant benzodiazepines in the last decade have been diazepam, lorazepam, alprazolam, temazepam, chlordiazepoxide, nitrazepam, triazolam, flunitrazepam, and lormetazepam.

In this chapter dealing with the chemistry, pharmacokinetics, and pharmacodynamics of benzodiazepines, we focus mainly on flunitrazepam (FN). FN was first introduced on the market in 1975, in Switzerland, under the trade name of Rohypnol®. It is indicated to treat insomnia and as a preoperative anesthetic. International sales data indicate that, over the past 10 yr, FN has accounted for an average of 6–7% of sales of sedative–hypnotics in 20 countries, including

From: *Forensic Science: Benzodiazepines and GHB: Detection and Pharmacology*
Edited by: S. J. Salamone © Humana Press Inc., Totowa, NJ

the major European markets, Japan, Australia, South Africa, Brazil, Venezuela, and Mexico, among others *(3)*. It has estimated worldwide sales of 2.3 million doses a day *(4)* but is not approved by the Food and Drug Administration (FDA) for use in the United States.

In recent years, the drug has been smuggled into the United States from Mexico and central and southern America for illegal use *(3,5,6)*. The first reported police seizure of FN was on June 15, 1989 in Miami, Florida *(5)*. In 1983, FN was classified as a Schedule IV drug by the U.N. Convention on Psychotropic Substances. Despite little evidence of abuse, it was the first benzodiazepine to be moved in March 1995 to Schedule III by the World Health Organization (WHO). This scheduling requires more rigid controls, and was based largely on reports that FN was involved in a high incidence of illicit activities and that it was widely abused by opioid addicts *(3,7)*. Its ability to cause euphoria and a drunk-like "high" is the likely reason for the increasing abuse of FN in recent years at parties, night clubs, and rave dances. Street names are numerous and include the following: roofies, rophies, rophynol, ruffies, roché, roches, roach, ropes, rib, reyna, the date-rape drug, and the forget pill *(5)*. In the United States it has also become a tool in drug-facilitated rapes. Mixture with alcoholic beverages results in unconsciousness, hypnosis, and amnesia of the rape victims *(3,4)*. In Europe the abuse of FN by ingestion, smoking, injection, or intranasal application is popular among heroin addicts. The rapid onset of sedation ("slowing down", "to be turned off") can ameliorate symptoms of opiate withdrawal, reducing stress, anxiety, or depression and can also enhance the effects of alcohol and cannabis *(3,8)*. There have been reports of abuse of FN in Florida, Texas, and other states *(5,9,10)*.

Those who have used lysergic acid diethylamide (LSD) or marijuana in the past or who have a peer or partner who used this drug appear to be at greater risk of abuse *(11)*. Doses and frequency of use vary from 1 to 15 tablets once or occasionnally twice a week. Habitual users frequently report ingesting FN with alcohol or in combination with cannabis *(5)*. In 1996, Customs regulations were changed, making it illegal to bring the medication across the U.S. border, and some states (like Florida, Oklahoma) have already classified FN as a Schedule I drug *(5,12)*.

2. CHEMISTRY

The classical benzodiazepines are based on a 5-aryl-1,4-benzodiazepine structure in which the benzene ring is linked to the 6–7 bond of the 1,4-diazepine (Figs. 1 and 2). The aryl substituent at position 5 is usually phenyl (e.g., oxazepam) or 2'-halophenyl (e.g., 2-fluorophenyl for flunitrazepam or 2-chloro-

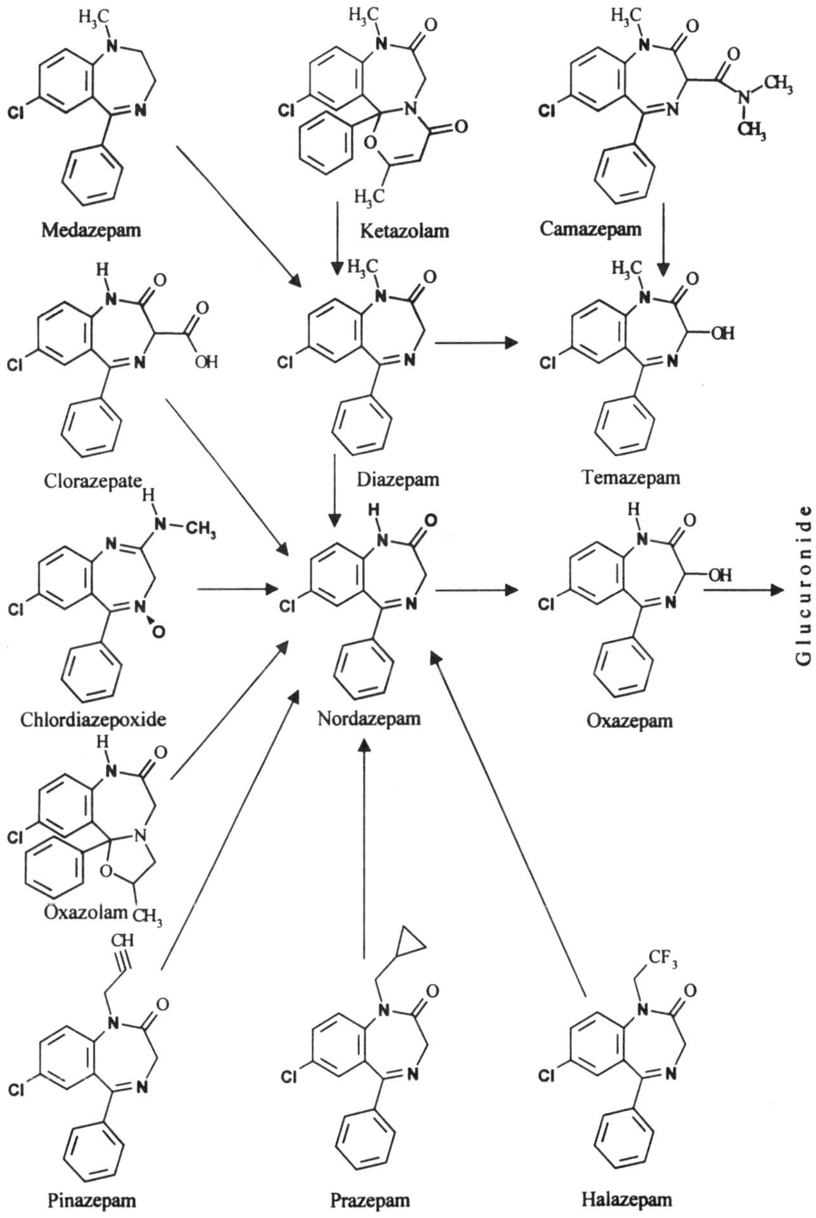

Fig. 1. General routes of metabolism for 1,4-benzodiazepines.

phenyl for lorazepam). The more recently introduced benzodiazepines include variations such as an imidazole (1,3-diazole) ring fused to the 1–2 bond of the 1,4-diazepine, that is, the imidazolobenzodiazepines, for example, midazolam

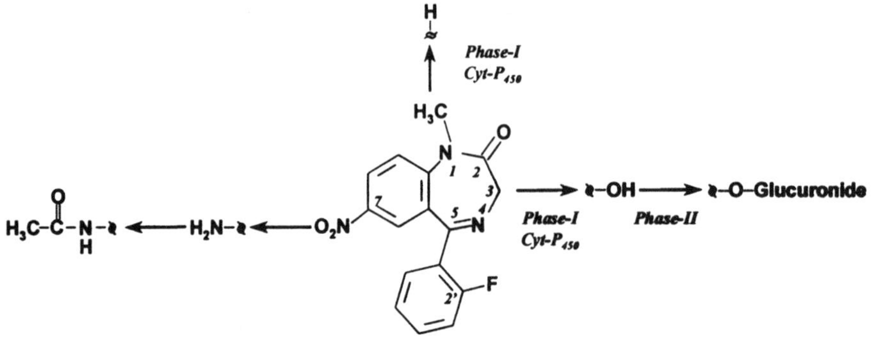

Flunitrazepam (INN); Rohypnol®
7-nitro-5-(2'-fluorophenyl)-1,3-dihydro-1-methyl-(2H)-1,4-benzodiazepine-2-one

$C_{16}H_{12}FN_3O_3$

m.wt. 313.3

CAS-no. 1622-62-4

pKa 1.82 [2,21]

Solubility in water 6.0 µg/ml (pH 7.4, 37°C) [14]

Fig. 2. Chemical characteristics and metabolic pathways of flunitrazepam.

(Fig. 3) or loprazolam. In a similar way, the triazolobenzodiazepines have a 1,2,4-triazole ring instead of the imidazole. Examples are alprazolam, estazolam and triazolam (Fig. 3). Other structural modifications include annelation of heterocyclic rings at the 4–5 bond, for example, haloxazolam, ketazolam, and oxazolam (Fig. 1) or replacement of the benzene ring by a thienyl ring (clotiazepam). Many benzodiazepines are hydrolyzed in acid solutions to form the corresponding benzophenone derivatives which can be used for analytical purposes. In the free base/acid form, benzodiazepines are generally soluble in most organic solvents such as ethyl ether, ethyl acetate, chloroform, and methanol, but are practically insoluble in water *(1)*.

3. PHARMACOKINETICS

3.1. Absorption, Distribution, and Plasma Levels

FN is administered orally or by intravenous or intramuscular injection in doses of 0.5–2 mg. FN is lipophilic at physiological pH and is absorbed very quickly and almost completely after oral administration: FN undergoes first-pass metabolism in the liver, resulting in a systemic bioavailability of 85–90%.

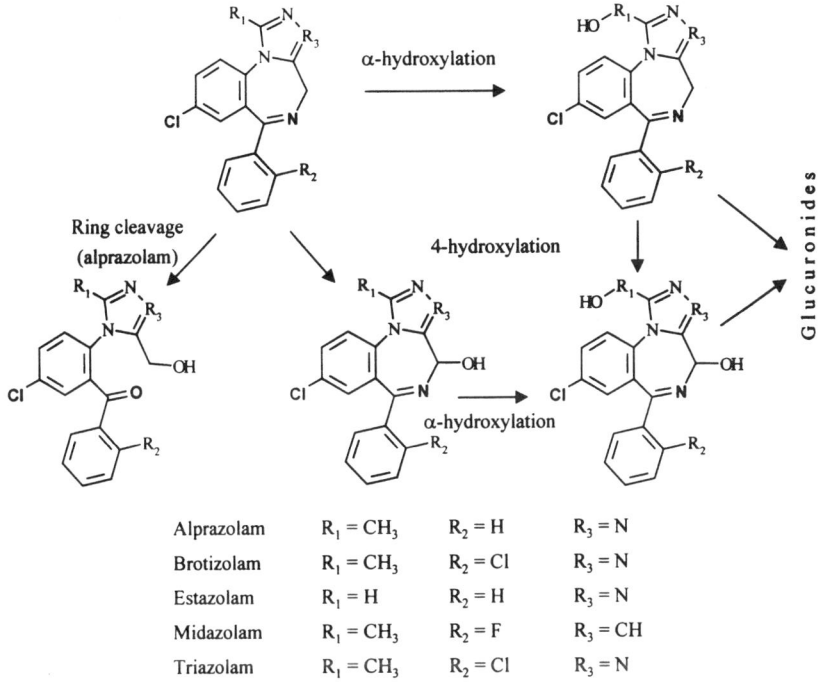

Fig. 3. General routes of metabolism for triazolo- and imidazobenzodiazepines.

The onset of action is directly linked to the absorption rate from the gastrointestinal tract, a fact that holds true for all benzodiazepines *(13)*.

The pharmacokinetic parameters of single- and multiple-dose oral FN are summarized in Table 1. FN absorption and disposition follow first-order kinetics after single- and multiple-dose oral administration *(14)*. The distribution is biphasic and lasts up to 20 h, with an initial half-life of 2–4 h. The rapid uptake into the brain is followed by a fairly rapid distribution out of the central compartment. Two-compartment models are in most cases adequate to describe the plasma concentration–time profiles of oral FN, whereas three-compartment models are used for intravenous FN *(15)*. After a single oral dose of 2 mg, plasma peaks of 8.8 ± 3.0 ng/mL FN occur 1.90 ± 1.38 h after administration *(16)*. A slight accumulation can be observed in plasma after subchronic to chronic administration. Steady-state occurs 3–5 d after administration (*N*-desmethyl-FN: 5–7 d) with a volume of distribution (V_{ss}) of 2.2–4.1 L/kg. The pharmacokinetic data of intravenous FN (mean dose 21 μg/kg, n = 12) based on a three-compartment open model are shown in Table 2 *(17)*. More than 95% of FN is bound to plasma proteins, with a blood-to-plasma ratio of 0.65–0.80 *(14)*. In a clinical study, where 2 mg of FN were administered orally, FN

Table 1
Pharmacokinetics of Oral Flunitrazepam (14–16,23,27,30,31)

Absorption	Fast, up to 100 %; $t_{1/2}$ = 0.17–0.5 h *(15)*; 0.14 h (2 mg, single dose), 1.14 h (0.5–2 mg, multiple doses) *(14)*
Bioavailability	85–90%; 10–15 % liver first-pass metabolism.
Plasma peaks	C_{max} = 8.8 ± 3.0 ng/mL (2 mg) *(16)*; 3.4–7.5 ng/mL (10 mg, blood) *(31)*; t_{max} = 0.5–2 h (1, 2, 4 mg) *(15)*; 1–1.5 h (0.5–1 mg) *(32)*; 1.90 ± 1.38 h (2 mg) *(16)*; 0.5–2 h (10 mg, blood) *(31)*
Plasma elimination half-life	$t_{1/2}$ = 20–30 h (FN), 10–16 h (7-amino-FN), 23–33 h (*N*-desmethyl-FN) *(30)*; 18.1 ± 11.8 h *(16)*; 13.5 h (2 mg, single dose), 19.2 h (0.5–2 mg, multiple doses) *(14)*
Distribution	V = 3.4–5.5 L/kg; V_{ss} = 2.2–4.1 L/kg *(30)*; V_{ss} 4.4 L/kg (2 mg, single dose), 6.6 L/kg (0.5–2 mg, multiple doses) *(14)*; V_{ss} = 162 L/kg (*N*-desmethyl-FN), 92 L/kg (7-amino-FN) *(15)*
Plasma protein binding	>95%
Blood-to-plasma ratio	0.75 (0.65–0.80) *(14)*
Plasma clearance	CL = 1.7–2.4 mL/min/kg *(30)*; 4.7 mL/min/kg (2 mg, single dose), 4.7 (0.5–2 mg, multiple doses) *(14)*; 60 mL/min (*N*-desmethyl-FN), 119 (7-amino-FN) *(15)*

was observed only in whole blood, whereas 7-amino-FN was present in both plasma and blood, with higher concentrations in plasma *(18)*. The time of detectability in blood is about 4 and 12 h for FN and 7-amino-FN, respectively.

The therapeutic plasma range of FN is 0.005–0.015 mg/L *(19)*. Maximum therapeutic serum drug levels are 0.020 mg/L for FN and 7-amino-FN *(1)*. Levels may exceed these during chronic therapy, in the elderly, in those with reduced liver or kidney function, and in patients for whom the dose is increased following the development of tolerance. Minimum levels for toxicity are 0.050 and 0.200 mg/L for FN and 7-amino-FN, respectively *(1)*. In forensic samples from drivers under the influence (DUI) of drugs FN can be present in serum at concentrations from 0 to 55 ng/mL *(20)*. The levels of 7-amino-FN, *N*-desmethyl-FN, and 3-hydroxy-FN ranged from 0 to 36, 0 to 36, and 0 to 12 ng/mL, respectively. Urine concentrations of 7-amino-FN ranged from 103 to 5777 ng/mL in 81 DUI cases collected in South Florida *(21)*. Urine specimens from volunteers ingesting 1–4 mg of flunitrazepam orally showed positive immunoassay results for up to 60 h, and metabolites could be detected by gas chromatography/mass spectrometry (GC/MS) beyond 72 h post-ingestion *(22)*.

Table 2
Pharmacokinetics of Intravenous Flunitrazepam (17)

Plasma elimination half-life	$t_{1/2}$ = 25 (FN)
Distribution	V = 3.6 L/kg
Plasma clearance	CL = 94 mL/min

3.2. Half-Life vs Duration of Action

Remarkable differences can be observed in the half-lives ($t_{1/2}$) of benzodiazepines; this is in contrast to the pharmacodynamic characteristics, which are similar for most benzodiazepines. Pharmacokinetic data can be the rational base for therapeutic use of benzodiazepines but also for forensic interpretations. Benzodiazepines can be classified according to their duration of action *(1)*:

- Short-acting benzodiazepines, half-life <10 h: brotizolam, clotiazepam, loprazolam, lorazepam, lormetazepam, midazolam, oxazepam, temazepam, triazolam.
- Intermediate-acting benzodiazepines, half-life 10–24 h: bromazepam, clonazepam, delorazepam, estazolam, flunitrazepam, tetrazepam.
- Long-acting benzodiazepines, half-life >24 h: chlordiazepoxide, clobazam, clorazepate, cloxazolam, diazepam, ethyl loflazepate, flurazepam, halazepam, ketazolam, medazepam, nitrazepam, nordazepam, pinazepam, prazepam, oxazolam.

It needs to be noted that the duration of action of certain benzodiazepines depends not only on the half-life of the drug itself, but also on the rate of metabolism, the formation of active metabolites, and the rates of distribution into and out of the brain *(3)*. In some cases the effect disappears long before the elimination phase is reached, as a result of redistribution of FN into body tissues *(23)*. Therefore the plasma elimination half-life contributes to, but is not the sole determinant of, the duration of action. Absorption half-life, distribution half-life, and dose are therefore better pharmacokinetic predictors *(24)*.

3.3. Metabolism and Excretion

Benzodiazepines are metabolized through a variety of oxidation such as hydroxylation (aliphatic and aromatic), desalkylation, or reduction reactions (phase I) followed in many cases by acetylation or glucuronidation (phase II) prior to excretion *(1)*. Often, the phase I metabolites have some degree of pharmacological activity, whereas the conjugates have no efficacy. The general routes of metabolism are shown in Figs. 1–3, based on the reviews in refs. *1* and *25*. Figure 1 illustrates the metabolic pathways for 1,4-benzodiazepines. Nordazepam and oxazepam (glucuronide) are common metabolites of several benzodiazepines. Figure 2 shows the metabolism of FN, which is representative for other 7-nitrobenzodiazepines (e.g., nitrazepam, nimetazepam, clonazepam) also. Nitrazepam in addition undergoes ring cleavage to the corresponding aminobenzophenone. The metabolism of triazolo- and imidazolobenzodiazepines is depicted in Fig. 3. It involves primarily hydroxylation at positions 1 and 4 as well as ring cleavage in the case of alprazolam to form the corresponding methylaminobenzophenone.

In humans FN is extensively metabolized through a variety of metabolic reactions (Fig. 2). These consist of $N(1)$-desmethylation, $C(3)$-hydroxylation followed by O-glucuronidation, and reduction of the nitro group to the amine with subsequent acetylation. In vitro experiments have shown that the desmethylation and hydroxylation steps are mediated by the cytochrome P_{450} isoenzymes CYP2C19, CYP3A4, and CYP1A2 *(26)*. Various combinations of biotransformation reactions are possible, and more than 12 metabolites are present in urine. The major ones include 7-amino-FN (10% of an oral dose), 3-hydroxy-FN (3.5%), 7-acetamido-nor-FN (2.6%), and 3-hydroxy-7-acetamido-FN (2%). Less than 0.2% of the drug is excreted unchanged *(1,4,27)*. Several metabolites have pharmacological activity, especially the N-desmethyl- *(15,28)*, the 7-acetamido-N-desmethyl-FN, and notably 7-amino-FN, which possesses anesthetic activities in animals *(23)*. Typically, an average of 84% of a radiolabeled dose is eliminated in the urine *(4)*. In a controlled clinical study administering single oral doses of 1 and 4 mg FN, 7-amino-FN was the most abundant metabolite in urine detectable up to 72 h after ingestion. 3-Hydroxy-FN was detected in only a few samples, whereas other FN metabolites and the parent drug could not be found *(29)*.

4. PHARMACODYNAMICS

4.1. Sites of Action

γ-Aminobutyric acid (GABA) is the most widely distributed inhibitory neurotransmitter in the human brain. GABA owes its pharmacology to at least three receptor subtypes: $GABA_{A-C}$. Whereas $GABA_A$ is coupled to a chloride channel (Fig. 4), $GABA_B$ is coupled to cationic channels (K^+, Ca^{2+}) via G-proteins and second-messenger systems, and $GABA_C$ are chloride channels with totally different pharmacology than $GABA_A$. A chloride channel allows negatively charged Cl^- ions to enter the neurons and lower the resting membrane potential (hyperpolarization), resulting in a less excitable tissue and decreased neuronal function. The three GABA receptors have distinct structures, distinct functions, and different cellular localization and pharmacology. $GABA_A$ receptors are made of five subunits, and each subunit spans the neuronal mem-

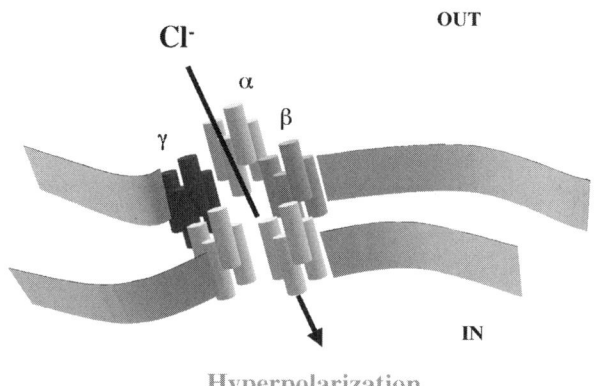

Fig. 4. General structure of a $GABA_A$ receptor.

branes four times. These subunits are chosen from a family of 6 α, 4 β, 4 γ, 1 δ, 1 ε, or 1 π. This complex stoichiometry can clearly give rise to several subtypes of $GABA_A$ receptors: the most abundant human CNS receptor type is the α1β2γ2 isoform. Classically, $GABA_A$ receptors have modulatory (allosteric) sites for the binding of benzodiazepines, barbiturates, and neurosteroids (Fig. 5).

The functional response of the channel to both GABA and to its modulators is dependent on the subunit composition of the receptor complex. Both α- and γ-subunits are necessary for benzodiazepine binding to the $GABA_A$ receptor. Whereas certain aminoacid residues of the α- and γ-subunits are critical for the binding of benzodiazepines, the γ-subunit type can also influence the efficacy (EC_{50}) of the benzodiazepines (33). Molecular studies have revealed interesting differences in the binding selectivity of benzodiazepines to subtypes of the $GABA_A$ receptor. These are the first insights into a possible different pharmacodynamic of benzodiazepines and will contradict the common notion that all benzodiazepines act in a similar manner and are different only through their respective pharmacokinetics. Pharmacological analysis has underlined the importance of phenylalanine and methionine at positions 77 and 130 on γ2-subunits: high-affinity binding of FN and other benzodiazepines such as clonazepam and triazolam requires Met130, whereas high-affinity binding of other ligands, such as flumazenil, depends more on Phe77 (34). Certain amino acid residues of the α-subunits are just as critical for FN binding, such as the histidine residue at position 102 (35). Allosteric regulation of FN binding by other GABA ligands, such as barbiturates, can depend on the subunit composition of the receptor: for example, α1γ2 receptor binding of FN is inhibited by pento-

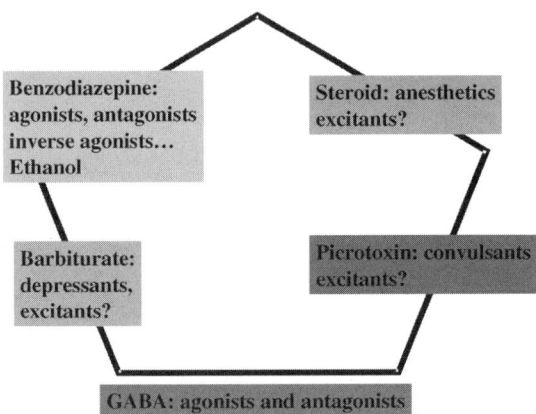

Fig. 5. Modulatory sites associated with the $GABA_A$ receptor.

barbital and etomidate, whereas $\alpha 1\beta 3\gamma 3$ binding is actually stimulated by the same compounds *(36)*. Even more disturbing is the report that FN can behave as an inverse agonist (thereby no longer causing sedation but insomnia, not causing anxiolysis but anxiety) on $\alpha 6\beta 2\gamma 2$ receptors *(37)*. This inverse agonist pharmacology could well explain the paradoxical effects of hyperactivity, insomnia, aggression, hallucinations, and anxiety sometimes seen with FN. It is these subtle differences that could explain why certain benzodiazepines, such as FN, may be more likely to be abused, or may cause a more powerful amnestic effect, a more potent anxiolysis, or a marked sedative effect. A better understanding of the subunit composition and brain region localization of the various $GABA_A$ subtypes will undoubtedly shed some light on pharmacodynamic differences between benzodiazepines.

4.2. Acute Effect

All benzodiazepines share to a certain extent the properties of potentiating GABA binding to its receptor and result in a certain degree of central nervous system (CNS) depression. This is clinically exhibited as a sedative, anxiolytic, and amnesic effect. High-potency benzodiazepines such as FN can be used as hypnotics to induce anesthesia and have a more pronounced anterograde amnesia effect. It is this action that is sought in the potential use of FN as a date-rape drug. An anterograde amnesia refers to a lack of memorization by the individual from the time of administration of the drug (parenteral) or after adequate absorption of the drug (oral). There is no change in previously memorized events (i.e., no retrograde amnesia). Small therapeutic doses of FN given intravenously or orally can clearly result in impaired memory; however, this effect is short lived and seems to decline rapidly within 30 min after administration of the drug *(23)*. The relatively short time window of the effect may be a reason for the small number of drug-facilitated rape associated with FN. To that effect, a study recently showed that out of 1179 samples collected from all states and Puerto Rico over a 26-mo period, only 97 were positive for benzodiazepines, including 6 for FN *(38)*. Enhancement of $GABA_A$ receptor function has been shown to disrupt the formation of memories in the hippocampal formation. The excitatory amino acid transmitters glutamate and aspartate are involved in plastic changes in neurons of this cerebral structures known as long-term potentiations (LTPs) involving the *N*-methyl-D-aspartate (NMDA) receptor. FN suppressed LTP induction and this effect was prevented by preadministration of the benzodiazepine receptor antagonist flumazenil *(39)*.

FN also has significant vasodilatory properties, and the relaxation of vascular smooth muscle with ensuing drop in blood pressure and reflexe increase in heart rate are quite specific to this drug. Diazepam is devoid of such an effect *(23)*. Drugs are sometimes abused owing to their vasodilatory properties: the draining of brain blood due to the pooling in dilated peripheral vessels is commonly understood as the reason for the abuse of nitrates ("poppers") and certain inhalants. It is possible that the cardiosuppressant effects of FN may add to the feeling of euphoria addicts report after the use of this drug. In a survey, "liking" scores for FN by heroin addicts were higher than for other benzodiazepines, and a clinical study has suggested that 2 mg of FN produces pleasurable feelings in healthy patients, a property not shared with another benzodiazepine, triazolam *(40)*.

1.3. Chronic Administration and Abuse Liability

The abuse liability of long-term treatment of benzodiazepines has been a concern. The risk of developing dependence using chronic therapeutic doses of these anxiolytics/sedatives occurs beyond 3–6 mo of treatment, and an abstinence syndrome is more likely the shorter the half-life of the drug administered (lorazepam more than diazepam or chlorazepate, for example). Katz et al. *(41)* have shown that drug-naïve subjects, in contrast to sedative abusers, did not experience significant reinforcing effects and may even have found drugs such as flurazepam and lorazepam aversive at moderate doses. Drug-naïve subjects could not discriminate between placebo and therapeutic doses of these benzodiazepines. Research has therefore shown that the recreational use of benzodiazepines is generally associated with subjects having histories of alcohol, methadone, or drug abuse. Even under these conditions, these abusers chose barbiturates over benzodiazepines *(42)*.

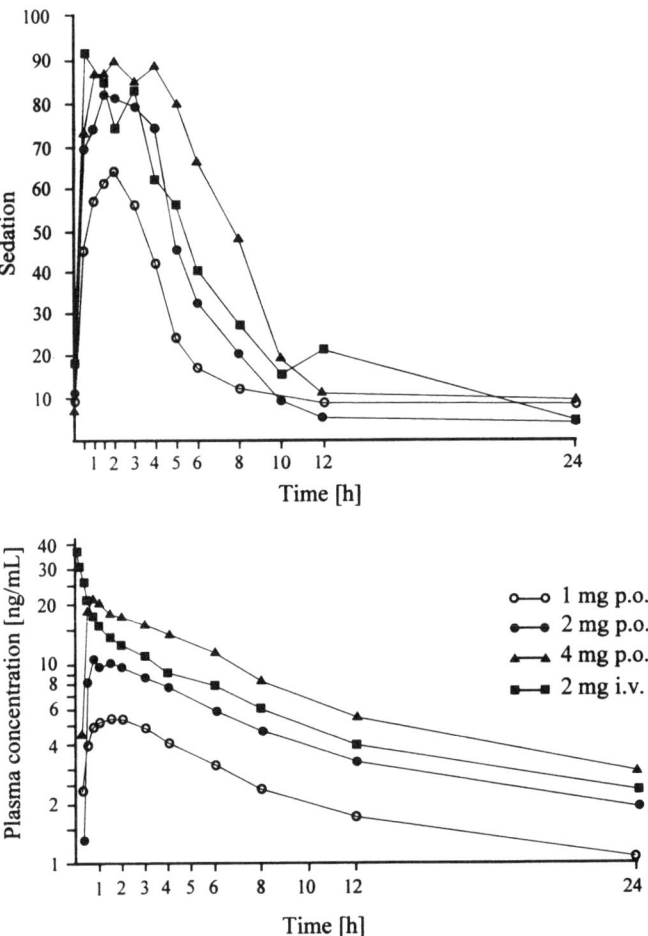

Fig. 6. Plasma levels of oral and intravenous FN vs sedative effects.

Withdrawal to benzodiazepines is characterized by rebound anxiety or insomnia, sometimes associated with headaches, nausea, vomiting, and muscle tremors. The symptoms are proportional to the duration of treatment and the abruptness of the cessation of use. Despite the lack of obvious dependence, benzodiazepines represent a potential of abuse: they are illegally traded as street drugs, are low cost, and can give symptoms reminiscent of opiates or alcohol to abusers of those drugs.

4.4. Pharmacokinetics vs Pharmacodynamics

As shown in Fig. 6, peak plasma concentrations of FN are reached within 0.5–2 h after a single oral dose of 1–4 mg FN, coinciding with the peak sedative

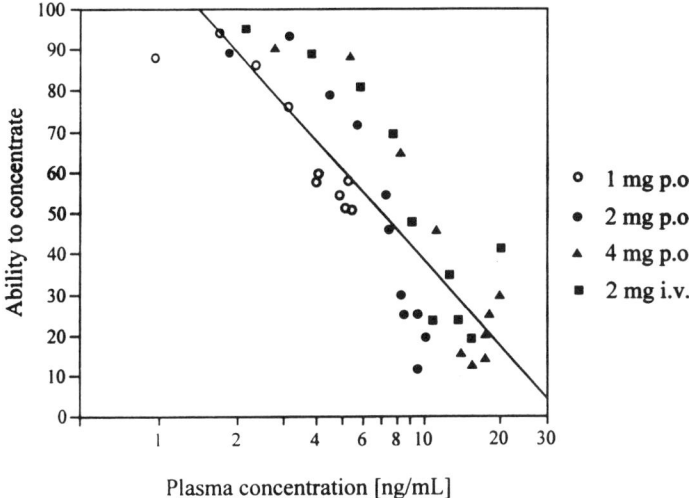

Fig. 7. Correlation between plasma concentration and ability to concentrate.

effect *(15)*. The correlation graph of plasma levels and the ability to concentrate after oral and intravenous administration of 1–4 mg FN is depicted in Fig. 7 *(43)*. In a recent study linear regression analysis of the relationship between plasma levels of FN and its effects indicated that there was a significant positive correlation between peak levels at night and impairment of night attention and explicit memory *(44)*. Threshold plasma levels exceeding 3–4 ng/mL FN are necessary to induce sedation, >7 ng/mL to impair performance, and 11–17 ng/mL to produce somnolence, strong sedation, and amnesia *(15)*.

4.5. Rohypnol®: The Debate

Awareness of the use of drugs as "chemical tools" to facilitate sexual assault has been highly publicized in the media in the recent years. Particular attention has focused on the use of Rohypnol® as a "date-rape" drug. By virtue of its sedative and anterograde amnestic effects, FN has been portrayed as a "drug of choice" in such criminal acts. Several studies have failed to confirm the widespread use of this benzodiazepine in drug-facilitated rape. Hindmarch and Brinkmann *(45)* showed that only six urine specimens out of 1033 samples collected from alleged rape victims were positive for FN. More importantly, alcohol and cannabinoids were present in close to 40% and 20% of these samples, respectively. Other benzodiazepines were present in more than 12% of the specimens analyzed. A similar study conducted by ElSohly and Salamone *(38)* essentially yielded the same data, with again six samples positive for FN out of 1179 specimens tested. Found much more often was alcohol, followed by cannabinoids and other benzodiazepines. FN may not be commonly used in drug-facilitated rape; however, significant abuse of the drug exists. FN has been reported as the most prevalent benzodiazepine confirmed in urine samples from DUI drivers in South Florida for several years and has been found in more than 10% of all DUI urine analyzed in Miami-Dade County in 1996 *(22)*. Rohypnol® is therefore more likely to be abused for its alcohol-like intoxicating effects by selected segments of the population, rather than used as a "date-rape" drug.

References

1. United Nations International Drug Control Programme (1997) *Recommended Methods for the Detection and Assay of Barbiturates and Benzodiazepines in Biological Specimens.* United Nations, New York.
2. Sternbach, L. H. (1979) The benzodiazepine story. *J. Med. Chem.* **22,** 1–7.
3. Woods, J. H. and Winger, G. (1997) Abuse liability of flunitrazepam. *J. Clin. Pharmacol.* **17,** 1S–57S.
4. Nguyen, H. and Nau, D. R. (2000) Rapid method for the solid-phase extraction and GC/MS analysis of flunitrazepam and its major metabolites in urine. *J. Anal. Toxicol.* **24,** 37–45.
5. Calhoun, S. R., Wesson, D. R., Galloway, G. P., and Smith, D. E. (1996) Abuse of flunitrazepam (Rohypnol) and other benzodiazepines in Austin and South Texas. *J. Psychoactive Drugs* **28,** 183–189.
6. Drug Enforcement Administration (DEA) (1995) Drug intelligence report—flunitrazepam (Rohypnol). *Microgram* **28,** 320.
7. World Health Organization (WHO) Expert Committee on Drug Dependence (1995) Twenty-ninth report. WHO Technical Report Series, No. 856, WHO, Geneva.
8. Ladewig, D. R., Hersberger, K., and Borner, S. (1995) Benzodiazepine in der Drogenszene. *Schweiz. Apoth. Ztg.* **133,** 319–322.
9. National Institute on Drug Abuse (1996*) Epidemiologic Trends in Drug Abuse,* Vol. I: *Highlights and Executive Summary.* NIH Publication No. 96-4128. National Institutes of Health, Rockville, MD.
10. Saum, C. A. and Inciardi, J. A. (1997) Rohypnol misuse in the United States. *Subst. Use Misuse* **32,** 723–731.
11. Rickert, V. I., Wiemann, C. M., and Berenson, A. B. (1999) Prevalence, patterns, and correlates of voluntary flunitrazepam use. *Pediatrics* **103,** E61–E65.
12. Rohypnol® was moved from Schedule IV to Schedule I (1997) in *Florida Statute* F.S. 893.03(1)(a).
13. Shader, R. I., Pary, R. J., Harmatz, J. S., Allison, S., Locniskar, A., and Greenblatt, D. J. (1984) Plasma concentrations and clinical effects after single oral doses of prazepam, chlorazepate and diazepam. *J. Clin. Psychiatry* **45,** 411–413.
14. Boxenbaum, H. G., Posmanter, H. N., Macasieb, T., Geitner, K. A., Weinfeld, R. E., Moore, J. D., et al. (1978) Pharmacokinetics of flunitrazepam following single- and

multiple-dose oral administration to healthy human subjects. *J. Pharmacokinet. Biopharmacol.* **6**, 283–293.
15. Crevoisier, C., Schoch, P., and Dingemanse, J. (1993) *Flunitrazepam (Rohypnol®, Ro 05-4200)—Monograph on Receptor Binding, Pharmacokinetics and Drug Effects.* Roche Research Report No. B-160 627, Hoffmann-La Roche, Basel.
16. Linnoila, M., Erwin, C. W., Brendle, A., and Logue, P. (1981) Effects of alcohol and flunitrazepam on mood and performance in healthy young men. *J. Clin. Pharmacol.* **21**, 430–435.
17. Kangas, L., Kanto, J., and Pakkanen, A. (1982) A pharmacokinetic and pharmacodynamic study of flunitrazepam. *Int. J. Clin. Pharmacol. Ther. Toxicol.* **20**, 585–588.
18. ElSohly, M. A., Feng, S., Salamone, S. J., and Brenneisen, R. (1999) GC-MS determination of flunitrazepam and its major metabolite in whole blood and plasma. *J. Anal. Toxicol.* **23**, 486–489.
19. Schütz, H. (1989) *Benzodiazepines II—A Handbook.* Springer-Verlag, Berlin.
20. Bogusz, M. J., Maier, R.-D., Krüger, K.-D., and Früchtnicht, W. (1998) Determination of flunitrazepam and its metabolites in blood by high-performance liquid chromatography-atmospheric pressure chemical ionization mass spectrometry. *J. Chromatogr. B* **713**, 361–369.
21. Raymon, L. P., Steele, B. W., and Walls, H. C. (1999) Benzodiazepines in Miami-Dade County, FL driving under the influence (DUI) cases from 1995-1998 with emphasis on Rohypnol®: GC/MS quantitation, patterns of use, psychomotor impairment, and results of Florida legislation. *J. Anal. Toxicol.* **23**, 490–499.
22. ElSohly, M. A., Feng S., Salamone, S. J., and Wu, R. (1997) A sensitive GC-MS procedure for the analysis of flunitrazepam and its metabolites in urine. *J. Anal. Toxicol.* **21**, 335–340.
23. Mattila, M. A. K. and Larni, H. M. (1980) Flunitrazepam: a review of its pharmacological properties and therapeutic use. *Drugs* **20**, 353–374.
24. Greenblatt, D. J. (1995) The pharmacology of benzodiazepines: comments on terminology and sources of data. *Psychopharmacology* **118**, 119.
25. Huang, W. and Moody, D. E. (1995) Immunoassay detection of benzodiazepines and benzodiazepine metabolites in blood. *J. Anal. Toxicol.* **19**, 333–342.
26. Coller, J. K., Somogyi, A. A., and Bochner, F. (1999) Flunitrazepam oxidative metabolism in human liver microsomes: involvement of CYP2C19 and CYP3A4. *Xenobiotica* **29**, 973–986.
27. Baselt, R. C. and Cravey, R. H. (eds.) (1995) *Disposition of Toxic Drugs and Chemicals in Man*, 4th edit., Chemical Toxicology Institute, Foster City, CA.
28. Berthault, F., Kintz, P., and Mangin, P. (1996) Simultaneous high-performance liquid chromatographic analysis of flunitrazepam and four metabolites in serum. *J. Chromatogr. B* **685**, 383–387.
29. Salamone, S. J., Honasoge, S., Brenner, C., McNally, A. J., Passarelli, J., Goc-Szkutnicka, K., et al. (1997) Flunitrazepam excretion patterns using the Abuscreen OnTrak and OnLine immunoassays: comparison with GC-MS. *J. Anal. Toxicol.* **21**, 341–345.
30. *Drugs Compendium of Switzerland 1998* (1997), 19th edit., Documed AG, Basel.
31. Winkler, M. B., Macasieb, T. C., and Wills, R. J. (1985) *Pilot Investigation of the Pharmacokinetic and Pharmacodynamic Interaction Between Flunitrazepam (Ro*

5-4200) and Ethanol: Pharmacokinetic Portion (Protocol 1053). Roche Research Report No. N-123603, Hoffmann-La Roche, Nutley, NJ.
32. Clarke, R. S. J., Dundee, J. W., McGowan, W. A. W., and Howard, P. J. (1980) Comparison of the subjective effects and plasma concentrations following oral and i.m. administration of flunitrazepam in volunteers. *Br. J. Anaesth.* **52,** 437–445.
33. Hadingham, K. L., Wafford, K. A., Thompson, S. A., Palmer, K. J., and Whiting, P. J. (1995) Expression and pharmacology of human $GABA_A$ receptors containing gamma 3 subunits. *Eur. J. Pharmacol.* **291,** 301–309.
34. Wingrove, P. B., Thompson, S. A., Wafford, K. A., and Whiting, P. J. (1997) Key aminoacids in the gamma subunit of the $GABA_A$ receptor that determine ligand binding and modulation at the benzodiazepine site. *Mol. Pharmacol.* **52,** 874–881.
35. Duncalfe, L. L., Carpenter, M. R., Smillie, L. B., Martin, I. L., and Dunn, S. M. (1996) The major site of photoaffinity labelling of the gamma-amino butyric acid type A receptor by (^{3}H)flunitrazepam is histidine 102 of the alpha subunit. *J. Biol. Chem.* **271,** 9209–9214.
36. Slany, A., Zezula, J., Fuchs, K., and Sieghart, W. (1995) Allosteric modulation of (^{3}H) Flunitrazepam binding to recombinant $GABA_A$ receptors. *Eur. J. Pharmacol.* **291,** 99–105.
37. Hauser, C. A., Wetzel, C. H., Berning, B., Gerner, F. M., and Rupprecht, R. (1997) Flunitrazepam has an inverse agonistic effect on recombinant $\alpha 6\beta 2\gamma 2$-$GABA_A$ receptors via flunitrazepam-binding site. *J. Biol. Chem.* **272,** 11,723–11,727.
38. ElSohly, M. A. and Salamone, J. A. (1999) Prevalence of drugs used in cases of alleged sexual assault. *J. Anal. Toxicol.* **23,** 141–146.
39. Seabrook, G. R., Easter, A., Dawson, G. R., and Bowery, B. J. (1997) Modulation of long term potentiation in CA1 region of mouse hippocampal brain slices by $GABA_A$ receptor benzodiazepine site ligands. *Neuropharmacology* **36,** 823–830.
40. Farre, M., Teran, M. T., and Cami, J. (1996) A comparison of the acute behavioral effects of flunitrazepam and triazolam in healthy volunteers. *Psychopharmacology* **125,** 1–12.
41. Katz, J. L., Winger, G. D., and Woods, J. H. (1991) Abuse liability of benzodiazepines and 5HT1A agonists, in *5HT1A Agonists, 5HT3 Antagonists and Benzodiazepines: Their Comparative Behavioural Pharmacology* (Rodgers, R. J. and Cooper, S. J., eds.), John Wiley & Sons, New York, pp. 317–341.
42. Woods, J. H., Katz, J. L., and Winger, G. D. (1992) Benzodiazepines, use, abuse, and consequences. *Pharmacol. Rev.* **44,** 151–347.
43. Amrein, R., Cano, J. P., Hartmann, D., Ziegler, W. H., and Dubuis, R. (1979) Clinical and psychometric effects of flunitrazepam observed during the day in relation to pharmacokinetic data, in *Sleep Research* (Priest, R. G., Pletscher, A., and Ward, J., eds.), MTP Press, Falcon House, Lancaster, U.K., pp. 83–98.
44. Bareggi, S. R., Ferini-Strambi, L., Pirola, R., and Smirne, S. (1998) Impairment of memory and plasma flunitrazepam levels. *Psychopharmacology* **140,** 157–163.
45. Hindmarch, I. and Brinkmann, R. (1999) Trends in the use of alcohol and other drugs in cases of sexual assaults. *Hum. Psychopharmacol. Clin. Exp.* **14,** 225–231.

Chapter 2
Immunoassay Detection of Benzodiazepines
Tamara N. St. Claire and Salvatore J. Salamone

1. INTRODUCTION

Benzodiazepines were first introduced in the 1960s as a safer alternative to phenobarbital. In the 1970s and mid-1980s, diazepam (Valium) was the most commonly prescribed benzodiazepine. The dose levels and excretion patterns of these first generation benzodiazepines produced concentrations in samples that made drug detection easy by immunoassay *(1)*. As chemists explored structure–activity relationships of this new class of compounds, a new generation of benzodiazepines was developed that exploited substituent activation of 1,4-benzodiazepine *(2)*. These new benzodiazepines therefore were more potent prescribed in lower doses. This new generation of benzodiazepines was also fast acting and had much shorter half-lives with respect to blood concentrations and excretion levels.

The higher doses and longer half-lives of the diazepam-related benzodiazepines, made it possible to detect this class of drugs by immunoassay screening. After a single dose of 5 mg of Valium, immunoassay detection is possible for up to 2 wk *(1)*. With the lower dose, faster clearing benzodiazepines, (alprazolam *[3]*, triazolam *[4]*, lorazepam *[5]*, nitrazepam *[6]*, flunitrazepam *[7]*, and clonazepam *[8]*), detection by immunoassay at historical cutoff levels was nearly impossible. Although most of the currently available immunoassays showed

From: *Forensic Science: Benzodiazepines and GHB: Detection and Pharmacology*
Edited by: S. J. Salamone © Humana Press Inc., Totowa, NJ

good cross-reactivity for the parent drug of these low-dose benzodiazepines, the pharmacokinetics of these drugs are such that very little parent drug appears in the urine; these drugs are extensively metabolized and conjugated with glucuronic acid *(9)*. These glucuronide conjugates are generally not crossreactive with the antibodies used in the instrument-based tests. Owing to the lower levels of drug that appear in the urine along with extensive glucuronidation, therapeutic doses of these drugs screen negative within a short time from ingestion.

As toxicologists sought consistency between laboratory results of known users of benzodiazepines, they explored the use of glucuronidases and lower cutoffs to increase immunoassay sensitivity. Manual procedures that were first developed added the enzyme in vast excess to the urine sample off-line *(10–13)*. The standard practice for many years was addition of glucuronidase from *Escherichia coli* or *Helix pomatia*, in 50% glycerol, directly to the sample without buffering. Incubation times for these hydrolysis procedures ranged from 1 hr to overnight. Incubation temperatures ranged from ambient temperature to 37°C. After the hydrolysis procedure, an aliquot of the pretreated sample was then placed on the clinical chemistry analyzer for analysis.

Manual procedures have evolved to where the glucuronidase is now added along with a buffer to the sample off-line to retain optimal enzyme activity. The concentration of enzyme used in these procedures is still high so as to compensate for the inhibitory effects of constituents in the large volume of urine used. These manual methods, although effective, require a great deal of enzyme, are labor intensive, and are sensitive to matrix effects from the relatively large volume of urine.

In the late 1990s, procedures were developed that utilized the automation of the clinical analyzer *(7,14)*. By placing the enzyme in a reagent or sample position on the analyzer, the instrument was programmed to deliver the enzyme to a cuvette that contained a sample diluted with the first reagent from the immunoassay kit. This procedure allowed for reduced consumption of the enzyme owing to the buffered environment and the small sample volume.

The immunoassay manufacturers have also responded to the laboratory's needs in several ways. Biosite Diagnostics, in the Triage™ product *(15)*, has developed antibodies with high cross-reactivity to the glucuronidated benzodiazepines. Microgenics has incorporated β-glucuronidase in the cloned enzyme donor immunoassay (CEDIA) immunoassay reagents *(16)*. Roche Diagnostics has developed a fluorescent polarization assay on the COBAS INTEGRA with a low cutoff (7 ng/mL in urine, 3 ng/mL in serum) and high cross-reactivity to the low-dose benzodiazepine drugs *(17)*. These reagents and procedures dramatically improve sensitivity and, depending on the purpose, may provide the toxicologist with the desired performance.

Immunoassay of Benzodiazepines

The objectives of this chapter are to provide background information on the use of β-glucuronidase treatment to guide the toxicologist on effective use of this enzyme. The utility of altering cutoff levels is discussed and general procedures are provided on how to use the glucuronidase treatment in both the manual and automated modes.

2. OPTIMAL ENZYME ACTIVITY

2.1. Conditions

A good understanding of the parameters affecting enzyme activity is vital in achieving maximum sensitivity for a benzodiazepine screening assay.

Previous studies have characterized conditions required to achieve optimal enzyme activity for the hydrolysis with β-glucuronidase *(18,19)*. The most recent study by Dou et al. *(19)*, determined binding constants of lorazepam–glucuronide, oxazepam–glucuronide, and temazepam–glucuronide. This study showed a difference in binding (K_m) and catalytic (K_{cat}) constants, using enzyme from the *E. coli* source, that were less than an order of magnitude under the same reaction conditions. In addition, the catalytic efficiency (K_{cat}/K_m) did not differ to a great extent, illustrating that all three benzodiazepine glucuronides would react similarly.

The pH and temperature profile along with optimal incubation times for the three glucuronides were also determined by Dou. The pH optimum for each of the substrates was shown to be between pH 6 and pH 7. The pH profile of enzyme activity is illustrated in Fig. 1. Dou's temperature study showed increased activity with increasing temperature, which is consistent with Meatherall's 1994 study *(18)*. Most clinical instruments use a 37°C incubation temperature; these studies illustrate that this temperature would be adequate for complete hydrolysis. Finally, studies on the incubation time showed the reaction was very rapid and reached a plateau within 15 min (Fig. 2). In applying this to the labor-atory, shorter incubation times can be achieved by using higher enzyme concentrations.

β-glucuronidase has been used in both manual and automated methods. The manual methods generally require addition of large amounts of enzyme to a relatively large volume of urine with or without buffer addition to stabilize the pH. The automated methods use a much smaller sample volume and are diluted with one of the immunoassay reagents. These conditions require a smaller quantity of enzyme. The advantages of using the automated method are: the enzyme is stabilized by the reagent diluent and the diluted sample minimizes potential sample matrix effects. In addition, the automated system has the advantage of faster throughput and less operator intervention.

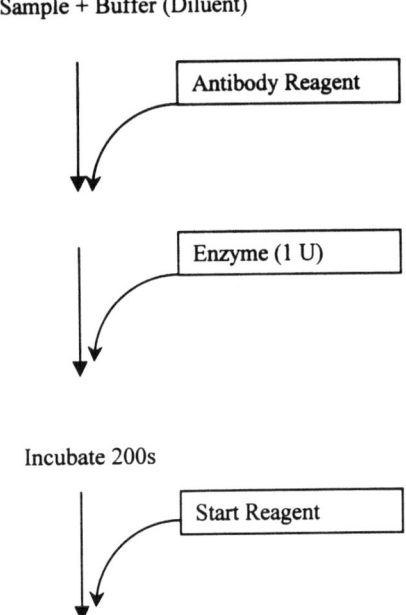

Fig. 1. pH profiles from 4.5 to 8.0 for the enzymatic hydrolysis of benzodiazepine conjugates in buffered urine.

Using the automated system with optimal enzyme conditions, where the pH is between 6 and 7, and incubation temperature is 37°C, the enzyme levels can be adjusted to shorten incubation times.

2.2. Activity

The activity of an enzyme is often described as an International Unit (U). One International Unit is the amount of enzyme, under standard conditions, that produces 1 µmol of product per minute (min). Assuming optimal activity, the required enzyme concentration for complete hydrolysis is minimal. For instance, the automated method described by Beck et al. *(14)* has a sample volume of 18 µL diluted into an R1 reagent of 77 µL. 1 U of β-glucuronidase is added and the mixture is incubated for 3.33 min (200 seconds) at 37°C on the COBAS MIRA.

The following exercise illustrates what 1 U of enzyme can catalyze in the above example:

$$1\ U = 1 \times 10^{-6}\ mol/min$$

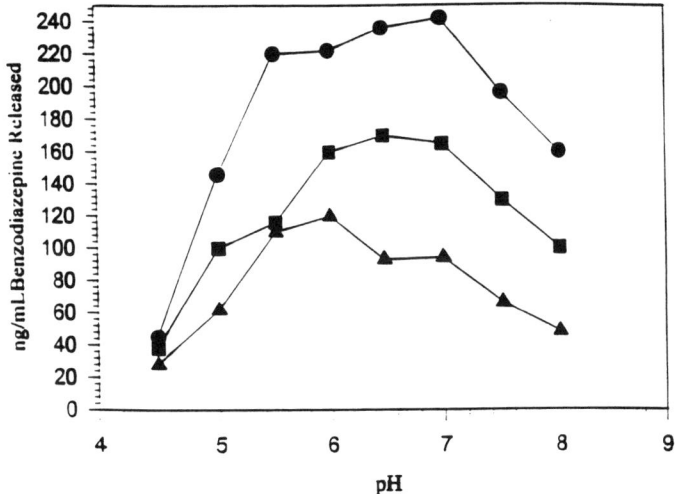

Fig. 2. The effect of incubation time on hydrolysis of benzodiazepine glucuronides. Note the reaction is very rapid within the first 15 minutes.

The approximate formula weight of a benzodiazepine–glucuronide (BG) is 500 g/mol.

Therefore 1 U of enzyme will convert:

1×10^{-6} mol/min $\times$ 500 g/mol = 5×10^{-4} g/min or 500,000 ng/min of BG

Considering that only 18 µL of sample was used, and the incubation time was 3.33 min, the following calculation represents the concentration (ng/mL) of glucuronidated benzodiazepine that can be converted in the COBAS application given above:

1000 µL/mL $\times$ 1/18 µL $\times$ 3.33 min $\times$ 500,000 ng/min = 9×10^7 ng/mL
or 90,000,000 ng/mL

This calculation demonstrates that merely 1 U of enzyme can convert a vast amount of glucuronidated benzodiazepine in a short period of time. Although 1 U of enzyme is in excess, this amount safely accounts for experimental variations. Most methods, either manual or automated, use far more than 1 U of enzyme, in many cases up to 5000 U. This excessive amount of enzyme represents an obvious undue expense to the laboratory.

The following generalized equation can be used to calculate the quantity of glucuronidated benzodiazepine hydrolyzed in different applications of the automated hydrolysis procedure:

$1/A \times B \times 5 \times 10^8$ = ng/mL of BG hydrolyzed where

A = μL sample per test
B = minutes of incubation time

To use this equation, the two unknowns must be inserted. The volume of sample added to the cuvette is variable A and the incubation time in minutes is variable B. If modifying an application, use the sample size (A) that is recommended by the manufacturer. Modifying sample size is an option in achieving optimal conditions; however, incubation time (B) is the variable that most laboratories adjust to achieve optimal enzyme hydrolysis. In optimizing a particular hydrolysis procedure, referring to the exercise above, one should aim to hydrolyze approximately 9×10^7 ng/mL of benzodiazepine–glucuronide (BG).

3. CUTOFF

Lowering the cutoff of an immunoassay in combination with sample hydrolysis with β-glucuronidase can assist in eliminating false-negative results. Consideration must be used in lowering the cutoff so as not to produce a greater number of false-positive results. This must be thoroughly controlled with validation and verification. Including proper controls during calibration will ensure that the new cutoff is above the limit of detection (LOD) of the assay.

To realize the increased sensitivity with hydrolysis in detecting single doses of low-dose benzodiazepines, the method must have a cutoff level that is lower than what has been traditionally used. Using a cutoff above 300 ng/mL to detect these low-dose benzodiazepines would have limited utility even if enzyme hydrolysis is utilized.

4. IMMUNOASSAYS

The following is an overview of the performance of the most widely used immunoassay screening methods and the effect of hydrolysis on the sensitivity of the methods. There are several widely marketed commercial products available to screen for benzodiazepines. Most techniques cannot reliably detect therapeutic doses of the new generation of benzodiazepines. The difference in performance between methods is mainly due to the different calibrators used and the difference in antibody cross-reactivities. The cross-reactivity is related to the antibody's immunoreactivity to the parent drug of each analyte as well as each metabolite present. It is important to remember that quantitative results must be interpreted with caution, as the calibrator may be a different drug than the analyte(s) detected.

The role of the calibrator on the performance of the method is related to both the cutoff and the characteristic binding curve of the analyte chosen for

Table 1
Immunoassay Sensitivity and Cutoff

Immunoassay	LOD	Cutoff
FPIA	40 ng/mL	200 ng/mL
EMIT	70 ng/mL	300 ng/mL
CEDIA	6.8 ng/mL	200 ng/mL
CEDIA	8.3 ng/mL	300 ng/mL
Online	5 ng/mL	100 ng/mL
SBENZ	7 ng/mL	7 ng/mL

the calibrator. The cutoff of an assay is based on the reactivity of the antibody to the drug used to calibrate the method. Each manufacturer claims a recommended cutoff and limit of detection based on the calibrator's performance. Table 1 shows the sensitivity (LOD) and cutoff claims for the commercial benzodiazepine immunoassays.

All benzodiazepines (and their metabolites) that are screened will have a relative cross-reactivity with respect to the calibrator. The cross-reactivity of each benzodiazepine may also vary with concentration, as the binding curve may not be parallel to the calibrator's binding curve. For example, the fluorescence polarization immunoassay (FPIA) on the Abbott ADx has a cross-reactivity for oxazepam of about 90% at the detection limit of 200 ng/mL nordiazepam, but at concentrations of oxazepam greater than 1 µg/mL, the cross-reactivity declines to less than 50% *(20)*. Table 2 demonstrates the cross-reactivities of several benzodiazepines for enzyme-multiplied immuno-technique (EMIT) and FPIA (TDx) determined by Meatherall *(18)*. Values are posted as the percentage of the screening result versus the drug concentration in the sample.

All automated methods have low cross-reactivity to the glucuronidated metabolites. At least 75% of the benzodiazepines that are excreted in urine are glucuronide conjugates *(21)*. Hydrolysis is generally required for most of the commercially available assays to ensure detection of these conjugated benzodiazepines. For example, lorazepam is excreted from the body primarily as a glucuronide metabolite *(22)* and cannot be detected by Online, EMIT, or FPIA without hydrolysis *(11)*.

Hydrolysis can have a varying effect on each commercial method owing to the difference in the selectivity of the antibody for the hydrolyzed and glucuronidated analyte. For example, pretreatment does not increase the sensitivity of FPIA or EMIT for flurazepam. The cross-reactivity for the glucuronidated flurazepam is high in the native systems. This can be explained by similar immunoreactivity for flurazepam and its glucuronide.

Table 2
Percent Cross-Reactivity of Benzodiazepine Metabolites

	Free drug					Conjugated drug (ng/mL)
	200 ng/mL	500 ng/mL	1000 ng/mL	2000 ng/mL	5000 ng/mL	
Oxazepam						
EMIT II	96	107	91	100	A[a]	0.2–22
TDx	66	57	46	34	26	0–13
Temazepam						
EMIT II	156	385	A	A	A	3
TDx	58	75	77	70	A	0
Nordiazepam						
EMIT II	200	A	A	A	A	700–3400
TDx	98	91	102	A	A	200–800
Lorazepam						
EMIT II	37	30	23	16	10	0.3–56
TDx	0	0	6	8	6	0–18
α-OH-alprazolam						
EMIT II	248	>400	A	A	A	45–833
TDx	82	84	82	75	A	24–140
α-OH-triazolam						
EMIT II	133	211	207	A	A	
TDx	30	37	31	21	21	
2-OH-ethylflurazepam						
EMIT II	191	>400	A	A	A	
TDx	57	75	76	65	A	
N-desalkyl-3-OH-flurazepam						
EMIT II	46	41	31	22	17	
TDx	5	23	24	19	13	

[a]Analyzed value above the highest calibrator (i.e., 2000 ng/mL for EMIT II or 2400 ng/mL for TDx). From ref. *12*.

Sample pretreatment with β-glucuronidase may also extend the window of detection for benzodiazepine drugs. In a clinical study using controlled doses of flunitrazepam, use of β-glucuronidase increased the positive rate and provided a longer period of detection after dosing *(13)*.

With improved sensitivity and a lower cutoff, a loss in specificity may be encountered. An appropriate confirmation method can compliment increased detection. It is important that the principal analytes and metabolites are accounted for with the confirmation method, or a sample may be misdiagnosed as a false-negative. This approach can rule out the apparent loss of specificity owing to the increased detection of analytes not detected by the less sensitive confirmation methods.

EMIT II uses oxazepam as the calibrator with a 200 ng/mL cutoff. Calibration curves are stable for 1 mo. Meatherall found in a 1994 study that the cross-reactivities of temazepam and nordiazepam were greater than that of the calibrator for this method *(12)*.

The cross-reactivity for the oxazepam glucuronide is stated as 0.1% *(23)*. Oxazepam is a principal metabolite for other common benzodiazepines *(4)*. The EMIT assay was shown to pick up therapeutic concentrations of alprazolam and chlordiazepoxide. The method detected triazolam within the first 12 h of dosing, but it did not detect flunitrazepam, nitrazepam, or lorazepam over the entire test interval *(11)*. Hydrolysis and a cutoff lowered to 100 ng/mL improved EMIT response to benzodiazepines *(14)*.

FPIA generally reveals a higher number of positive results from sample pools used in comparative studies, largely because of the lower limit of detection *(10)*. FPIA on the Abbott TDx is calibrated with nordiazepam. The unmodified FPIA assay can generally detect therapeutic doses of alprazolam, flurazepam, and chlordiazepoxide. Flunitrazepam, oxazepam, lorazepam, nitrazepam, and triazolam require hydrolysis and a lower cutoff to improve detection rates *(11)*.

Beck found that hydrolysis increased the FPIA response for all benzodiazepines studied. With pretreatment, an oxazepam dose as low as 2.5 mg/dL could be detected *(10)*.

Microgenics has developed a new CEDIA reagent kit that incorporates β-glucuronidase in the reagent. In a study by Meatherall, CEDIA was evaluated by comparing the new CEDIA reagent, the original CEDIA reagent with off-line hydrolysis, CEDIA reagent without hydrolysis, EMIT II with off-line hydrolysis, and EMIT II without hydrolysis. In this study, without hydrolysis the original CEDIA kit failed to detect any positive samples. The new CEDIA reagent kit showed greater sensitivity than the original kit. It was able to identify a high number of positive samples. The CEDIA kit with the incorporated glucuronidase was also shown to detect a 1-mg dose of lorazepam equally as well as the off-line hydrolysis procedure *(16)*.

OnLine from Roche Diagnostics has three available cutoffs: 300 ng/mL, 200 ng/mL, and 100 ng/mL. The method uses nordiazepam as calibrator. A study using 50 random samples collected from drug users showed an 85% increase in sensitivity for the Online assay with enzyme hydrolysis *(14)*. Table 3 illustrates the increased positive rate with hydrolysis and demonstrates the

Table 3
Comparison of Different Cutoff Limits
Using the OnLine System with
and without Enzyme Hydrolysis

Online cutoff (ng/mL)	Positive rate (%)	
	No hydrolysis	With hydrolysis
100	68	90
200	58	84
300	48	68

The study was done with 50 patient samples that were positive for benzodiazepines with routine FPIA screening (14).

effect of different cutoffs in this study. An additional study (7), in which subjects were administered low doses of flunitrazepam, indicated using an automated hydrolysis procedure increased the immunoassay values by 20–80%. The OnLine glucuronidase applications can be easily adapted to the automated clinical analyzers, and Roche Diagnostics has applications for both the COBAS INTEGRA and Hitachi systems.

Table 4 compares the sensitivities of several benzodiazepine screening assays by type of drug found by gas chromatography/mass spectroscopy (GC/MS) in patient samples (14). Note the increase in positive results with hydrolysis, particularly for the OnLine assay. The high rate of positive values for analyte concentrations above 300 ng/mL for all assays is also noteworthy.

The urine-based Cassette COBAS INTEGRA Serum Benzodiazepine assay (SBENZ) from Roche Diagnostics is a new fluorescence polarization immunoassay using a nordiazepam calibrator with a 7 ng/mL LOD with a reported standard curve stability of 16 wk. Using a 7 ng/mL cutoff level, the sensitivity of the assay is high enough not to require enzyme hydrolysis. Sensitivity was reported to be equal to GC/MS (100%); specificity is reported as 71% vs GC/MS (17). This assay was also shown to be as sensitive as GC/MS in detecting single doses of flunitrazepam (24). With a 7 ng/mL cutoff level, this method represents the most sensitive immunoassay for the screening of benzodiazepines.

The SBENZ assay also has a serum application with a 3 ng/mL cutoff. This cutoff has been shown to be very effective in detecting low levels of low-dose benzodiazepines (14). In one study, single doses of flunitrazepam were detected over a 72-h period in serum and the clinical sensitivity was shown to be similar to GC/MS (14). In addition, a second calibration is not required when the matrix is changed from urine to serum or saliva (10).

Table 4
Comparison of Screening Methods for the Detection of Benzodiazepines

	7-Amino-flunitrazepam		7-Amino-nitrazepam		Oxazepam, nordiazepam, temazepam		Multicomponents	
	% positive	N	% positive	N	% positive	N	% positive	N
Concentration > 300 ng/mL								
FPIA[a] (modified)	69	13	100	4	100	11	100	3
Online	31	13	75	4	27	11	66	3
Online[a]	54	13	75	4	73	11	66	3
EMIT II	62	13	100	4	100	11	66	3
EMIT II[a]	100	11	66	3	100	8	100	3
EMIT d.a.u.	46	13	100	4	73	11	66	3
Concentration > 300 ng/mL								
FPIA[a] (modified)	90	20	91	11	100	39	100	13
Online	90	20	73	11	92	39	85	13
Online[a]	95	20	82	11	97	39	100	13
EMIT II	100	13	91	11	95	39	100	13
EMIT II[a]	100	13	100	8	97	35	100	6
EMIT d.a.u.	100	13	73	11	95	39	100	13

[a]With enzyme hydrolysis.
Applied with 100-ng/mL cutoff. All samples contained benzodiazepines or metabolites according to GC-MS.
From ref. *14*.

5. METHODS

5.1. Manual β-Glucuronidase Treatment

The following procedure describes the manual glucuronidase treatment of a urine sample for the detection of benzodiazepines. The resultant hydrolyzed mixture can be applied to any standard analyzer and evaluated by the FPIA, EMIT, CEDIA, or Online methods.

β-Glucuronidase (β-D-glucuronide glucuronosohydrolase, EC 3.2.1.31) from *E. coli* can be obtained from Roche. It is available as a 50% glycerol–water solution and is used without any additional treatment.

To a 1000-µL urine sample, add 50 µL of a 2 M phosphate buffer solution, pH 6.0, and vortex-mix thoroughly. To a 200-µL aliquot of the buffered urine sample, add 4 U of the enzyme preparation. (This should result in less than a 1.1-fold dilution.) Incubate the mixture at ambient temperature for 30 min. Load the hydrolysate as sample into the system for analysis. Calibrators and controls should be treated in the same manner as the sample for consistency and to account for procedural variations. Lowering the cutoff of the immunochemical method, closer to the limit of detection, will further increase the clinical sensitivity.

5.2. Automated β-Glucuronidase Treatment

Toxicologists have adapted the enzyme hydrolysis procedure for the benzodiazepine assay directly to the clinical analyzer. The automated procedure affords faster and easier analysis and uses lower levels of enzyme. In addition, a comparative study between manual and automated hydrolysis revealed that the automated method yielded higher clinical sensitivity, which was attributed to more effective hydrolysis *(8)*. The following illustrates two proven procedures for adapting commercial benzodiazepine reagents to an automated hydrolysis procedure followed by the illustration of a general scheme to assist in the broader adaptation of benzodiazepine reagents to the programmable clinical chemistry analyzer.

5.2.1. Online with the Hitachi 717

An optimized procedure that allows β-glucuronidase treatment with the Online reagent on the Hitachi 717 requires no changes to the instrument parameters—no additional cycles are required for incubation. The modified program utilizes glucuronidase from *E. coli* without further dilution. β-Glucuronidase is added directly to the benzodiazepine R1 in the amount of 28 µL of enzyme to 1 mL of reagent (or 5 mL of enzyme to the total R1). During the analysis, the sample is added to R1 at time zero and the mixture is incubated for 5 min. It is recommended that R1 containing enzyme be used within 24 h for best results.

5.2.2. Online with the COBAS INTEGRA 700

β-Glucuronidase from *E. coli* is added as a special diluent while programming the pipetting parameters. All of the test definitions remain the same. The unmodified application requires 10 µL of diluent (H_2O), which follows sample dispensing. In the hydrolysis application, the diluent (H_2O) volume is reduced to 8 µL to accommodate 2 µL of the special diluent (0.4 U of glucuronidase) that follows. Roche Diagnostics makes the procedure available in its Benzodiazepine Optional Applications insert.

5.2.3. A General Scheme

Beck presented an automated procedure for EMIT and Online reagents on the COBAS MIRA Plus. This automated approach can be applied with any set of immunological reagents to any programmable analyzer that has the ability to pipet an additional reagent.

There are several points to consider during optimization. Incubation Time: In order to optimize the system, procure fresh samples and try several different incubation times to determine if the hydrolysis has reached completion. In general, the time between addition of enzyme and start reagent is greater than 60 s. This time period is more than sufficient to hydrolyze the conjugated benzodiazepines. *Enzyme Levels*: Initially aim for the addition of 1 U of enzyme. To optimize enzyme levels, explore increasing enzyme concentration. For example, run the samples incubated with 1, 5, and 10 U of β-glucuronidase. When the recovery reaches a plateau, the enzyme level is adequate. Figure 3 illustrates the general approach to developing an automated enzyme hydrolysis procedure.

6. CONCLUSION

Most immunoassay systems lack sufficient sensitivity to screen for the commonly used benzodiazepines. All commercial immunoassay methods appear appropriate for screening with the addition of enzymatic hydrolysis. Toxicologists have the choice of performing manual or automated sample pretreatment depending on the desired performance and procedural commitment. Manual or automated hydrolysis is not only easily adaptable to assay procedures, but pretreatment has also been shown not to interfere with the benzodiazepine assay. Drug-free urine that was treated with enzyme showed readings below the lower limit of detection for both FPIA and EMIT, demonstrating that the hydrolysis procedure does not interfere with the assay performance *(4)*. The hydrolysis procedure was also found not to interfere with other drugs of abuse assays or the clinical chemistry creatinine assay *(4)*.

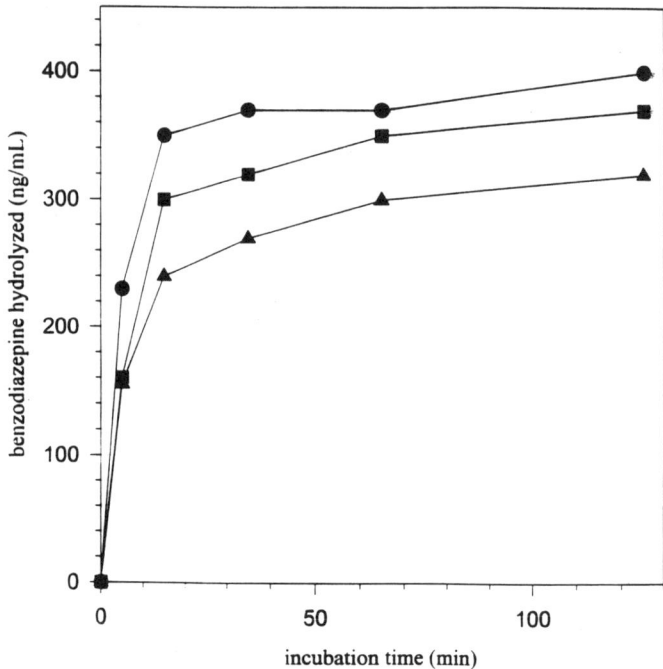

Fig. 3. A general scheme for the adaptation of hydrolysis on a programmable clinical analyzer.

References

1. Kaplan, S. A, Jack, M. L., Alexander, K., and Weinfeld, R. E. (1973) Pharmacokinetic profile of diazepam in man following single intravenous and oral and chronic oral administrations. *J. Pharmaceut. Sci.* **62,** 1789–1796.
2. Sternbach, L. H. (1973) Chemistry of the 1,4-benzodiazepines and some aspects of the structure-activity relationship, in *The Benzodiazepines* (Garattini, S., Mussini, E., and Randall, L. O., eds.), Raven Press, New York.
3. Dawson, G. W., Jue, S. G., and Brogden, R. N. (1984) Alprazolam: a review of its pharmacodynamic properties and efficacy in the treatment of anxiety and depression. *Drugs* **27,** 132–147.
4. Baktir, G., Fisch, H. U., Huguenin, P., and Bircher, J. (1983) Triazolam concentration-effect relationships in healthy subjects. *Clin. Pharmacol. Ther.* **34,** 195–201.
5. Greenblatt, D. J., Schillings, R. T., and Hyriakopoulos, A. A. (1976) Clinical pharmacokinetics of lorazepam. I. Absorption and disposition of oral ^{14}C-lorazepam. *Clin. Pharmacol. Ther.* **20,** 329–341.
6. Rieder, J. and Wendt, G. (1973) Pharmacokinetics and metabolism of the hypnotic nitrazepam, in *The Benzodiazepines* (Garattini, S., Mussini, E., and Randall, L.O., eds.), Raven Press, New York.

7. Salamone, S. J., Honasoge, S., Brenner, C., McNally, A. J., Passarelli, J., Goc-Szkutnicka, K., et al. (1997) Flunitrazepam excretion patterns using the Abuscreen Ontrak and Online immunoassays: comparison with GC-MS. *J. Analyt. Toxicol.* **21,** 341–345.
8. Berlin, A. and Dahlstrom, H. (1975) Pharmacokinetics of the anticonvulsant drug clonazepam evaluated from single oral and intravenous doses and by repeated oral administration. *Eur. J. Clin. Pharmacol.* **9,** 155–159.
9. Kaplan, S. A. and Jack, M. L. (1983) Metabolism of the benzodiazepines: pharmacokinetic and pharmacodynamic considerations, in *The Benzodiazepines: From Molecular Biology to Clinical Practice* (Costa, E., ed.), Raven Press, New York.
10. Beck, O., Lafolie, P., Odelius, G., and Boréus, L. (1990) Immunological screening of benzodiazepines in urine: improved detection of oxazepam intake. *Toxicol. Lett.* **52,** 7–14.
11. Beck, O., Lafolie, P., Hjemdahl, P., Borg, S., Odelius, G., and Wirbing, P. (1992) Detection of benzodiazepine intake in therapeutic doses by immunanalysis of urine: two techniques evaluated and modified for improved performance. *Clin. Chem.* **38,** 271–275.
12. Meatherall, R. (1994) Benzodiazepine screening using EMIT II and TDx: urine hydrolysis pretreatment required. *J. Analyt. Toxicol.* **18,** 385–390.
13. Simonsson, P., Liden, A., and Lindberg, S. (1995) Effect of β-glucuronidase on urinary benzodiazepine concentration determined by fluorescence polarization immunoassay. *Clin. Chem.* **41,** 920–923.
14. Beck, O., Lin, Z., Brodin, K., Borg, S., and Hjemdahl, P. (1997) The online screening technique for urinary benzodiazepines: comparison with EMIT, FPIA, and GC-MS. *J. Analyt. Toxicol.* **21,** 554–557.
15. Wu, A. H. B., Wong, S. S., Johnson, K. G., et al. (1993) Evaluation of the Triage system for emergency drugs-of-abuse testing in urine. *J. Analyt. Toxicol.* **17,** 241–245.
16. SOFT (1997) Poster #35 Enhanced sensitivity for the CEDIA dau benzodiazepine screening assay. Salt Lake City, UT.
17. Schwenzer, K. S., Pearlman, R., Tsilimidos, M., Salamone, S. J., Cannon, R. C., Gock, S. B., and Wong, S. H. Y. (2001) New fluorescence polarization immunoassays for analysis of barbituates and benzodiazepines in serum and urine: performance characteristics. *J. Analyt. Toxicol.* **24,** 726–732.
18. Meatherall, R. (1994) Optimal enzymatic hydrolysis of urinary benzodiazepine conjugates. *J. Analyt. Toxicol.* **18,** 382–384.
19. Dou, C., Bournique, J. S., Zinda, M. K., Gnezda, M., McNally, A. J., and Salamone, S. J. (2001) Comparison of the rates of hydrolysis of lorazepam-glucuronide, oxazepam-glucuronide and temazepam-glucuronide catalyzed by *E. coli.* β-D-glucuronidase using the online benzodiazepine screening immunoassay on the Roche/Hitachi 917 analyzer. *J. Forensic Sci.* **46,** 335–340.
20. Abbott Laboratories (1987) Product bulletin for TDx benzodiazepines, June 1987. Abbott Park, IL.
21. Baselt, R. C. and Cravey, R. H. (1995) *Disposition of Toxic Drugs and Chemicals in Man*, 4th edit., Chemical Toxicology Institute, Foster City, CA, pp. 432–433.
22. Greenblatt, D. J., Joyce, T. H., Comer, W. H., et al. (1977) Clinical pharmacokinetics of lorazepam: II. Intramuscular injection. *Clin. Pharmacol. Ther.* **21,** 220–230.
23. Chang, J. (1985) Comment to the editor. *Clin. Chem.* **31,** 152.
24. SOFT (1998) Workshop #7 Rohypnol Detection. Albuquerque, NM.

Chapter 3

Analysis of Flunitrazepam and Its Metabolites in Biological Specimens

Mahmoud A. ElSohly and Shixia Feng

1. Introduction

Flunitrazepam, 5-(2-fluorophenyl)-1,3-dihydro-1-methyl-7-nitro-2H-1,4-benzodiazepin-2-one, also commonly known as Rohypnol or "roofies," belongs to a highly potent group of benzodiazepines used mainly as hypnotic, sleeping aid, or preanesthetic agents (1–3). The drug is distributed in 80 countries throughout the world; however, it has never been approved for medicinal use in the United States. It is at present listed as a Schedule IV controlled substance under current U.S. statutes. The drug is smuggled into the United States across the Mexican border or from South American countries through Miami. It is alleged to have been involved in date-rape cases in the 1990s (4–8).

The detection of flunitrazepam and its metabolites in biological specimens is difficult as compared to older generation of benzodiazepines. The drug is extensively metabolized (9,10) through reduction of the 7-nitro group to produce 7-amino-flunitrazepam, followed by N-acetylation, N-1-demethylation, or hydroxylation at the C-3 position, followed by glucuronidation. The

From: *Forensic Science: Benzodiazepines and GHB: Detection and Pharmacology*
Edited by: S. J. Salamone © Humana Press Inc., Totowa, NJ

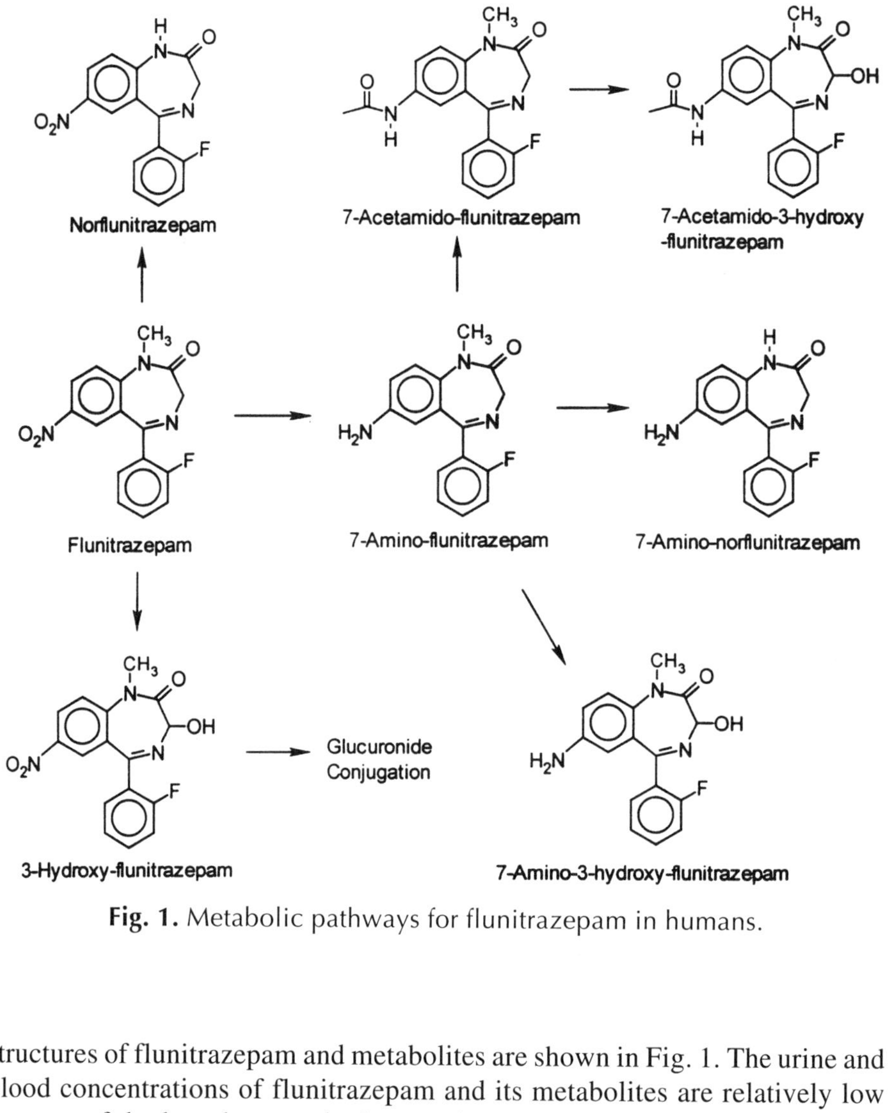

Fig. 1. Metabolic pathways for flunitrazepam in humans.

structures of flunitrazepam and metabolites are shown in Fig. 1. The urine and blood concentrations of flunitrazepam and its metabolites are relatively low because of the low therapeutic dosage (0.5–2 mg), extensive biotransformation, and high volume of distribution.

Numerous methods are currently available for determination of flunitrazepam and its metabolites in various biological specimens, such as urine, blood, and hair. Immunoassays, thin-layer chromatography, and gas and liquid chromatography with various detection methods have been described in the literature *(11–31)*. This chapter focuses on the recent developments as presented in the literature from 1991 through 2000.

2. Methods of Analysis

2.1. Screening Methods

Many commercial screening kits including enzyme multiple immunoassay tests (EMIT, Behring Diagnostic, San Jose, CA), fluorescence polarization immunoassay (FPIA, Abbott Labs, Abbott Park, IL), OnLine and OnTrak Immunoassay (both from Roche Diagnostic, Indianapolis, IN), and MicroPlate Enzyme Immunoassay (STC Technologies, Bethlehem, PA) have been evaluated as potential analysis methods for screening various biological specimens for flunitrazepam and its metabolites. Overall, the sensitivities of these screening methods are low and the application of these assays for determination of flunitrazepam often leads to false-negative results.

Flunitrazepam and its metabolites are reported *(13)* to react weakly with EMIT antibody. The cross-reactivity of flunitrazepam is only 60% relative to oxazepam at 300 ng/mL, and the cross-reactivity of 7-amino-flunitrazepam, the major metabolite in urine or blood, is not reported or not stated at all. Beck et al. *(13)* evaluated a procedure using 300 ng/mL as the cutoff value with oxazepam as a standard. In this procedure, 0.2 mL of urine sample was enzymatically hydrolyzed with 4 U of β-glucuronidase from *Escherichia coli* (β-D-glucoronide glucuronohydrolase, EC 3.2.1.31, from Boehringer Mannheim, Indianapolis, IN). Flunitrazepam intake produced a positive response in only one of six subjects during a 12–32-h interval who received a 1-mg single dose of flunitrazepam. The applicability of EMIT for flunitrazepam was recently reinvestigated by Morland and Smith-Kielland *(14)*. They reported that 100 out of 122 authentic urine specimens (80%) containing 7-amino-flunitrazepam had results above cutoff (200 ng/mL), and all samples had EMIT results different from zero. The sensitivity was improved when a lowered cutoff level was used (60 ng/mL). It was claimed that the risk of overlooking positive samples with EMIT cutoff at 60 ng/mL was negligible when an authentic urine control specimen containing ~60 ng/mL of 7-amino-flunitrazepam was included in the batch.

Flunitrazepam and its metabolites have also low cross-reactivity in FPIA systems, with 50% for flunitrazepam, 19% for 7-amino-flunitrazepam, 30% for norflunitrazepam, and 19% for 3-hydroxy-flunitrazepam relative to nordiazepam at 100 ng/mL. Beck et al. *(13)* evaluated two procedures using the FPIA method: enzymatically hydrolyzed or unhydrolyzed, both at a cutoff level of 100 ng/mL with nordiazepam as the standard substance. The procedure using hydrolysis step with 4 U of β-glucuronidase had increased sensitivity. It was able to produce three positive response out of six subjects during a 12–24-h interval who received a 1-mg single dose of flunitrazepam. In contrast, the unhydrolyzed procedure failed to detect any positive samples.

Table 1
Cross-Reactivity of Flunitrazepam
and Its Metabolites Relative to 100 ng/mL
of Nordiazepam in the OnLine and OnTrak Immunoassays

Compounds	OnLine	OnTrak
Flunitrazepam	55%	80%
7-Amino-flunitrazepam	30%	80%
3-Hydroxy-flunitrazepam	26%	27%
Norflunitrazepam	59%	59%
7-Amino-3-hydroxy-flunitrazepam	11%	20%
7-Amino-norflunitrazepam	10%	50%

Salamone et al. *(10)* compared the flunitrazepam excretion patterns using the Abuscreen OnTrak and OnLine Immunoassays (both from Roche Diagnostic System). The cross-reactivity of flunitrazepam and its metabolites in the OnLine and OnTrak immunoassays relative to 50 and 100 ng/mL of nordiazepam, respectively, is shown in Table 1.

The OnLine immunoassay reportedly has a clinical limit of detection of 26 ng/mL for urine, both with and without β-glucuronidase (0.4 U) treatment. The OnLine assay was run using a four-point linear curve based on nordiazepam (10, 50, 100, and 200 ng/mL) calibrators. The use of β-glucuronidase treatment improves the detectability of flunitrazepam use. The data showed that with the 1-mg dose, the urine concentration was below the clinical limit of detection. Using the enzyme hydrolysis pretreatment for 2.6 min, several samples showed low concentrations of cross-reactive benzodiazepines with the values ranging between 34 and 43 ng/mL and were found between 12 and 48 h.

The OnTrak assay is a single test qualitative assay with a 100 ng/mL cutoff using nordiazepam as a standard without enzyme hydrolysis. Because the OnTrak antibody has a higher cross-reactivity to flunitrazepam and metabolites than did the OnLine antibody, the OnTrak assay could identify all the OnLine samples that had values above 30 ng/mL as positive even without enzyme hydrolysis.

Recently, Negrusz et al. *(15)* reported the use of Micro-Plate Enzyme Immunoassay (STC Technologies, Bethlehem, PA) to screen flunitrazepam in hair. Although the kit itself is targeted at oxazepam, the assay was very sensitive (0.1 ng/mg cutoff) owing to the high cross-reactivity of 7-amino-flunitrazepam (156% oxazepam equivalent).

A highly sensitive and specific radioimmunoassay (RIA) with limit of detection of <0.1 ng/g for flunitrazepam in blood has been described by West et al. *(32)*. Flunitrazepam was derivatized in position 3 of the benzodiazepine ring to a coupling hapten that was coupled to a carrier protein. The flunitrazepam antibody was obtained by immunization of rabbits with this immunogen. The antibody showed a very sensitive and specific reaction with flunitrazepam and hardly any cross-reactivity to any other 1,4-bezodiazepines including the metabolites of flunitrazepam when tested in a heterogeneous, competitive RIA. However, because the urinary excretion of unchanged flunitrazepam is <1%, it is not a useful urine drug screening method.

Recently, Walshe et al. *(16)* reported a very sensitive and selective immunoassay for flunitrazepam and metabolites in urine that is based on the enzyme-linked immunosorbent assay (ELISA). In this procedure, sheep antiflunitrazepam antibody was coated on 96-well plates. When urine samples are added to the wells, flunitrazepam and its metabolites present in the sample will link to the antibody of the plates. Further addition of 7-amino-flunitrazepam linked to horseradish peroxidase (HRP) will result in a covalently bound complex (anti-flunitrazepam antiboby–flunitrazepam [or metabolites]-7-amino-flunitrazepam–HRP). The degree of antibody–flunitrazepam–HRP binding is therefore inversely proportional to the amount of drug in the sample. The assay is specific only to flunitrazepam and its metabolites with percentage cross-reactivity of 100%, 116.8%, 98%, 0.6%, and 56.8% for 7-amino-flunitrazepam, 7-acetamino-flunitrazepam, norflunitrazepam, 3-hydroxy-flunitrazepam, and flunitrazepam, respectively. Of 13 other benzodiazepines tested, diazepam was the only one that showed a significant degree of cross-reactivity (27.45%). The lowest level of 7-amino-flunitrazepam that could be reliably detected was 5 ng/mL. The urine samples from subjects taken from a 0.5–4-mg dose orally were analyzed by ELISA. At a 0.5-mg dose, flunitrazepam and/or cross-reactive metabolites were detected for up to 70 h after ingestion. With doses of 1 mg or above, the detection window was extended to up to 1 week.

2.2. HPLC Analysis

Numerous high-performance liquid chromatography (HPLC) procedures for determination of benzodiazepines including flunitrazepam and its metabolites have been reported. Usually, sufficient resolution can be achieved by HPLC; moreover, the mild working conditions are particularly suitable for labile compounds such as flunitrazepam. This section discusses several important issues associated with the HPLC method development for analysis of flunitrazepam and its metabolites.

2.2.1. Internal Standards

The highest precision and accuracy for quantitative chromatographic analysis can be obtained by using internal standard calibration because the uncertainty associated with the injection volume is minimized. For the HPLC procedures using ultraviolet (UV), diode array detection (DAD), or fluorescence detectors, the internal standards are differentiated from the analytes by retention time. Therefore, structurally similar benzodiazepines have been used as internal standards, because these compounds are sufficiently separated from the flunitrazepam and/or metabolites and yet close enough to the peaks of interest. For HPLC procedures using mass spectrometers as detectors, the most ideal internal standards are the isotopically labeled analogs of the analytes. These have identical physical properties to the actual analytes and therefore variations due to extraction efficiency and injection volume can be avoided. Such internal standards can be differentiated from the analytes by selected ion monitoring. Deuterium-labeled analogs that have been used for HPLC/MS include d_3-flunitrazepam and d_3-7-amino-flunitrazepam. Figure 2 shows the structures of these internal standards.

2.2.2. Extraction

Flunitrazepam and its metabolites must be separated from biological matrices before analysis can be conducted. The reported extraction procedures included liquid–liquid extraction, solid-phase extraction, and immunoaffinity extraction. Flunitrazepam is less polar and more lipophilic than its 7-amino-, N-desmethyl-, and 3-hydroxy metabolites. When using liquid–liquid extraction procedures for urine or blood specimens, greatest recoveries can be achieved if pH is adjusted to 9–9.5 using either borate buffer or ammonium hydroxide *(33)*. If extracted at a strong alkaline pH (0.1 M–1.0 M NaOH), the recoveries dropped dramatically. This was probably because the nitro group undergoes reduction followed by dimerization to form azo and azoxy derivatives *(34)*. Boukhabza et al. *(33)* reported that diethyl ether-methylene chloride (2:1, v/v) was better than chloroform for blood samples because it produced emulsion-free extracts (86% recovery for flunitrazepam and norflunitrazepam) with less interference. Berthault et al. *(35)* reported the use of diethyl ether–chloroform (8:2, v/v) to extract the serum samples after the pH was adjusted to 9.5 with ammonium hydroxide. The recoveries for flunitrazepam, 7-amino-flunitrazepam, 3-hydroxy-flunitrazepam, norflunitrazepam, and 7-amino-norflunitrazepam were 83%, 30%, 81%, 57%, and 83%, respectively. Difference in extraction efficiency could be attributed to the difference in polarity of these compounds. The use of other solvents such as methyl t-butyl ether (MTBE) or diethyl ether have also been reported *(36–38)*. For example, Darius and Banditt *(36)* reported the analysis of flunitrazepam in serum using liquid extraction with MTBE and by HPLC/APCI/MS/MS with an ion trap detector. Although the method was highly sensitive (limit of detection [LOD] = 0.19 ng/mL), no extraction recovery data were reported.

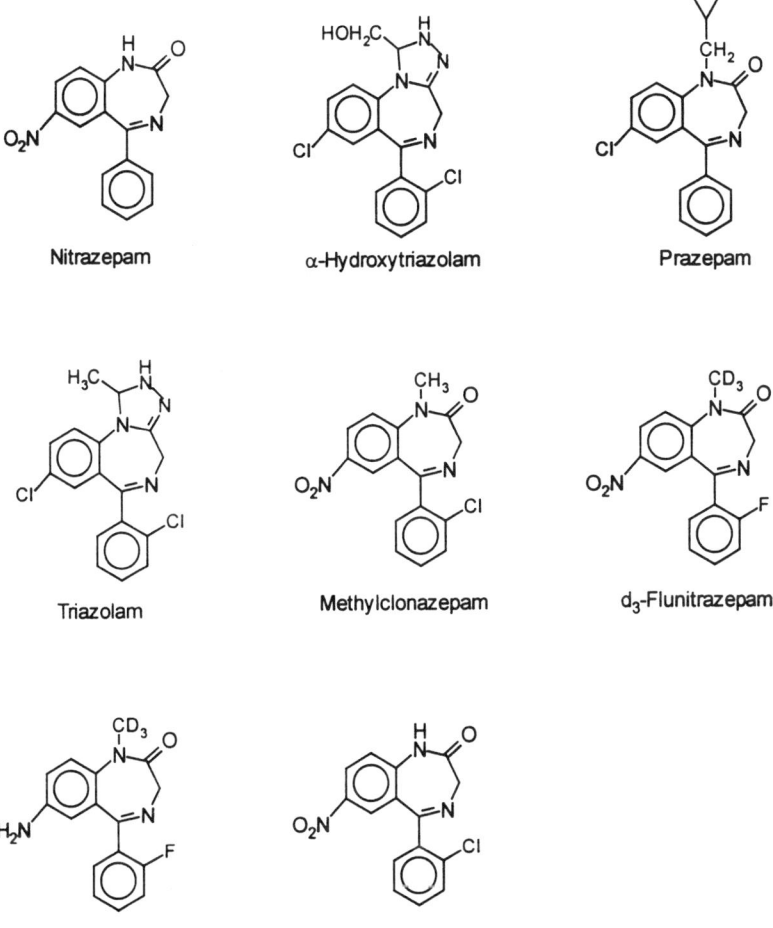

Fig. 2. Structures of some commonly used internal standards in HPLC analysis of flunitrazepam and metabolites.

Solid-phase extraction (SPE) methods have been gaining more favor over traditional liquid–liquid extraction over last decade. The advantages of SPE are known to be rapidity, reproducibility, ability to obtain cleaner extracts by using different washing solvents, and high recovery *(39,40)*. The retention mechanisms of SPE may be hydrophobic, polar, ionic, or mixed mode. The choice of these different types is based on the chemical properties of the analytes as well as the matrices. Nonpolar hydrophobic or mixed mode types SPE cartridges are often employed in the analysis of flunitrazepam and its metabolites.

When using SPE cartridges with a nonpolar sorbent, such as Sep-Pak C18, Bond Elute, and SuperClean C18, the urine or plasma samples are usually adjusted to pH 9.5–11 by the addition of a buffer solution such as ammonium carbonate before the sample is passed through the preconditioned SPE cartridges. These nonpolar sorbents with hydrophobic retention characteristics usually allow only a water-based wash step. The organic modifiers in the wash fluid will lead to lower recovery. Flunitrazepam and its metabolites are often eluted with organic solvents such as methanol, chloroform, acetonitrile, among others, or a mixture of these solvents. He and Parissis *(41)* reported the use of Sep-Pak C8 SPE cartridge to extract flunitrazepam and five metabolites, including 7-amino-norflunitrazepam, 7-acetamido-flunitrazepam, 7-amino-flunitrazepam, norflunitrazepam, and 3-hydroxy-flunitrazepam, from plasma and urine. The samples were enzymatically hydrolyzed with β-glucronidase (EC 3.2.1.31 G0876) from Sigma (St. Louis, MO) before extraction. The recoveries from urine ranged from 64% for 3-hydroxy-flunitrazepam to 99% for norflunitrazepam. However, for plasma, in which 77–80% of the absorbed flunitrazepam is bound to plasma proteins *(42)*, the recoveries were dramatically increased to 72–97% if the proteins were removed by precipitation with acetonitrile, as compared to 36–65% without protein precipitation. However, the necessity of the enzyme hydrolysis step has been questioned by a recent study *(43)* in which it was found that the concentrations of 7-amino-flunitrazepam, the major metabolite in blood and urine, does not change with or without enzyme hydrolysis. In fact, protein precipitation appeared to be an unnecessary step for other authors. Guichard et al. *(44)* reported an 89% recovery for flunitrazepam from human plasma, and Bogusz et al. *(45)* reported 93, 92, 99, and 96% recoveries for flunitrazepam, 7-amino-flunitrazepam, norflunitrazepam, and 3-hydroxyflunitrazepam, respectively. Both reports did not involve enzyme hydrolysis or protein precipitation steps.

The mixed mode SPE cartridges such as Bond Elute Certify® has been successfully used in the determination of flunitrazepam, 7-amino-flunitrazepam, 7-acetamido-flunitrazepam, and norflunitrazepam in urine and serum *(46)*. Bond Elute Certify® phase contains both nonpolar C8 sorbent and strong cation-exchange groups. Since flunitrazepam exhibits only weakly basic function (pK_a = 1.8), a highly acidic wash (pH 1.0) was needed to retain flunitrazepam on the SPE column. This cation-exchange property allows methanol and chloroform wash steps, which provide an efficient clean-up and result in much cleaner extracts and enhanced sensitivity. Elution was then achieved after switching the pH on column using chloroform–isopropanol–ammonia (78:28:2) as elution mixture. The recoveries for flunitrazepam, 7-amino-flunitrazepam, 7-acetamido-flunitrazepam, and norflunitrazepam ranged from 90% to 98% both at low and high concentrations.

Deinl et al. *(47,48)* reported the use of an on-line immunoaffinity column (IAC) for extraction of flunitrazepam, 7-amino-flunitrazepam, 7-acetamido-flunitrazepam, and norflunitrazepam in urine or serum. The IAC was packed with immunoaffinity sorbent which was prepared from polyclonal antibody raised against benzodiazepines and immobilized on glutardialdehyde-activated sorbent. The immunoaffinity sorbent had a capacity of 1200 ng of flunitrazepam. The apparatus included an IAC column, a preconcentration column, an analytical column, three pumps, and a tandem-switching valve. The sample was injected into the system and pumped through the IAC for 10 min by the first pump. After switching the tandem-switching valve, 90% methanol was pumped through the IAC for 10 min by a second pump, allowing the desorption of the analytes that were trapped on the preconcentration column. Finally, after switching the tandem-switching valve, the analytes were separated on the analytical column by the third pump. The recoveries were above 90% for all analytes.

2.2.3. HPLC Conditions

Reversed phase analytical columns with C8, C18, and cyano sorbents and guard columns with the same type of sorbent are frequently used for HPLC analysis of flunitrazepam and metabolites. Most reported procedures are capable of separating a number of structurally similar compounds if appropriate mobile phases are used. One study reported *(33)* the use of Nova Pak C18 (5 µm, 150 mm × 4.6 mm internal diameter [i.d.]) eluted with acetonitrile–methanol–6 mM phosphate buffer (23:13:64, v/v) at flow rate of 1.3 mL/min to separate flunitrazepam from 10 other benzodiazepines, including bromazepam, oxazepam, clonazepam, lorazepam, chlordiazeoxide, alprazolam, loflazepate, tofizopam, clobazam, and diazepam. Another study reported *(38)* the use of Nova Pak phenyl column (5 µm, 150 mm × 4.6 mm i.d.) to separate 15 related benzodiazepines and selected metabolites including 7-amino-flunitrazepam and flunitrazepam with a gradient mobile phase system. Deinl et al. *(45)* reported the use of 250 mm × 4.6 mm i.d. Lichrospher 60 RP-Select B (5 µm, Muller, Fridofing, Germany) to separate flunitrazepam, 7-amino-flunitrazepam, 7-acetamido-flunitrazepam, and norflunitrazepam from 16 other benzodiazepines within a run time of less than 20 min. An isocratic mobile phase system was used that contains acetonitrile–0.02 M phosphate buffer (pH 2.0, 36:64, v/v) at a flow rate of 1.0 mL/min. With slight modification *(46)*, the method was used to separate flunitrazepam and metabolites from methaqulone, chinine, and 12 other benzodiazepines. With a ChromSpher C8 column, a gradient mobile phase system containing methanol and 0.125% (v/v) of isopropyl amine in water was used to analyze flunitrazepam, 7-amino-norflunitrazepam, 7-amino-flunitrazepam, 7-acetamido-flunitrazepam, norflunitrazepam, 3-hydroxy-flunitrazepam, and 7-amino-3-hydroxy-flunitrazepam with triazolam as internal standard *(41)*.

2.2.4. Detection

UV detection is still the most widely used detection method. From LOD of 5–10 ng/mL in many early procedures to LOD of 1 ng/mL, the detection sensitivity for flunitrazepam has been largely improved over the last decade. Berthault et al. *(35)* reported the detection of flunitrazepam and four metabolites (7-amino-flunitrazepam, norflunitrazepam, 7-amino-norflunitrazepam, and 3-hydroxy-flunitrazepam) in serum at 242 nm wavelength with a liquid–liquid extraction procedure and prazepam as internal standard. The limit of detection ranged from 2.5–5.0 ng/mL and limit of quantitation (LOQ) was 10 ng/mL for each analyte. An efficient extraction procedure will result in clean extracts and clear chromatographic background, and hence improve the detection sensitivity. Such examples included the use of on-line immunoaffinity extraction and Bond Elute Certify® mixed-mode SPE cartridges. In these studies, a wavelength of 254 nm was used, and the limit of detection was 1 ng/mL urine or serum for flunitrazepam, 7-amino-flunitrazepam, 7-acetamido-flunitrazepam, and norflunitrazepam. These methods showed good precision and accuracy at both therapeutic and toxic concentrations *(45–47)*.

Questionable specificity is the weak point of HPLC with UV detection. HPLC with DAD is considered as a highly effective screening method. Criterion for identification of the analyte is that the maximum absorption wavelength in the UV spectrum of the analyte should be the same as that of the standard material within a margin determined by the resolution of the photo detection system, which for DAD is typically within ± 2 nm. The use of DAD gives the advantage of identifying the analyte both by retention time and the whole UV spectrum. In a reported procedure *(41)* using HPLC/DAD for determination of flunitrazepam and metabolites, the DAD was carried out at a monitoring wavelength of 240 nm and a reference wavelength of 550 nm. The LOD for flunitrazepam and five metabolites—7-amino-norflunitrazepam, 7-acetamido-flunitrazepam, 7-amino-flunitrazepam, norflunitrazepam, and 3-hydroxy-flunitrazepam—ranged from 1.42 to 5.3 ng/mL, and the LOQ ranged from 6.41 to 16.81 ng/mL in urine. 7-Acetamido-3-hydroxyflunitrazepam has very weak UV absorption at 240 nm; a more sensitive wavelength has to be selected for quantitation, that is, 248 nm.

Recent advances in interfacing of HPLC systems with mass spectrometers has provided a new dimension to therapeutic drug monitoring and forensic applications. The high sensitivity and specificity of mass spectrometry and the separation power of HPLC have made it possible to detect drugs such as flunitrazepam and its metabolites in biological specimens at very low concentrations. One study by Bogusz et al. *(45)* reported the use of solid-phase extraction and liquid chromatography (LC)-atmospheric pressure chemical ionization (APCI)/MS to determine flunitrazepam, 7-amino-flunitrazepam, norflunitrazepam, and 3-hydroxy-flunitrazepam in blood with d_3-flunitrazepam and d_3-7-amino-flunitrazepam as internal standards. The method used a single quadrupole instrument with selected ion monitoring (SIM). The SIM ions were selected from full scan LC/APCI/MS spectra of each analyte that were taken at octapole offset value of 40 V in positive ionization which caused distinct ion fragmentation by collision-induced dissociation (CID). The following ions were monitored: *m/z* 284 for 7-amino-flunitrazepam and flunitrazepam, *m/z* 287 for d_3-7-amino-flunitrazepam and d_3-flunitrazepam, *m/z* 300 for norflunitrazepam and 3-hydroxy-flunitrazepam, *m/z* 314 for flunitrazepam, and *m/z* 317 for d_3-flunitrazepam. The quantitative analysis of flunitrazepam, norflunitrazepam, and 3-hydroxy-flunitrazepam was performed against d_3-flunitrazepam as internal standard. The chromatographic conditions included a 125 mm × 3 mm Supersher RP C18 column (4 µm particle size) with an isocratic mobile phase system containing acetonitrile–50 mM ammonium formate buffer (pH 3.0, 45:55, v/v) at a flow rate of 0.3 mL/min. All peaks were resolved within 3–7 min. The limits of detection for flunitrazepam, 7-amino-flunitrazepam, norflunitrazepam, and 3-hydroxy-flunitrazepam were 0.2, 0.2, 1.0, 1.0 ng/mL, respectively, with linearity ranging from 1 to 500 ng/mL. It was reported that the use of APCI interface led to a sevenfold increase in sensitivity when compared to the electrospray ionization (ESI) method.

Darius and Banditt *(36)* recently reported the analysis of flunitrazepam in serum using HPLC/APCI/tandem-MS with an ion trap mass detector. The procedure employed a liquid–liquid extraction with clonazepam as internal standard. In the MS-MS experiments, the ions monitored for quantitation were the protonated product ions at *m/z* 268 for flunitrazepam and *m/z* 270 for clonazepam corresponding to the loss of their nitro groups [M + H − 46]$^+$. The LOD was found to be 0.19 ng/mL and LOQ was 0.5 ng/mL. This method showed good accuracy and reproducibility. The signal-to-noise ratio at 0.2 ng/mL was about 7:1 for flunitrazepam as compared to a signal-to-noise ratio of 3:1 by Bogusz et al.'s method *(45)*.

2.3. GC/MS Methods

Although numerous analytical procedures for analysis of flunitrazepam and its metabolites including GC/ECD, TLC, HPLC, especially the recent

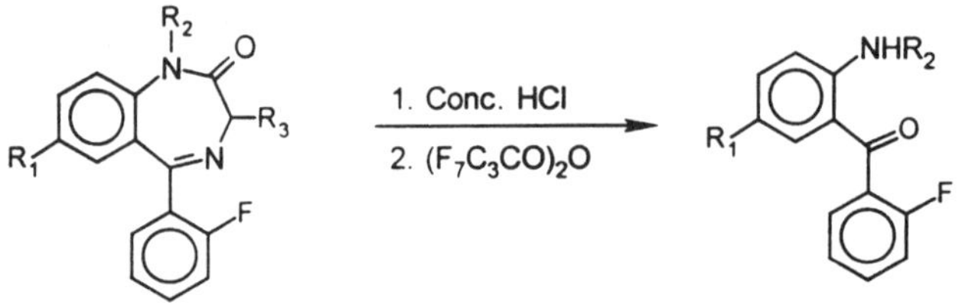

Fig. 3. Hydrolysis and derivatization of flunitrazepam and its metabolites.

$R_1 = NO_2$, $R_2 = CH_3$, $R_3 = H$ or OH
$R_1 = NO_2$, $R_2 = H$, $R_3 = H$ or OH
$R_1 = NH_2$ or $NHAc$, $R_2 = CH_3$, $R_3 = H$ or OH
$R_1 = NH_2$ or $NHAc$, $R_2 = H$, $R_3 = H$ or OH

1 $R_1 = NO_2$, $R_2 = CH_3$
2 $R_1 = NO_2$, $R_2 = NHCOC_3F_7$
3 $R_1 = NHCOC_3F_7$, $R_2 = N(CH_3)COC_3F_7$
4 $R_1 = NHCOC_3F_7$, $R_2 = NHCOC_3F_7$

development of LC/MS methods, GC/MS remains to be the main instrument in most drug testing laboratories today. The development of suitable GC/MS methods has become one of the important topics in recent literature of forensic toxicology.

The first reported GC/MS method for the analysis of flunitrazepam and its metabolites was based on acid hydrolysis of urine samples, which converts several related metabolites to benzophenones followed by conversion to heptafluorobutyrates (Fig. 3) and analysis of the latter *(49)*. Table 2 shows possible precursors to each of the four hydrolysis and derivatization products (**1–4**) analyzed. Two critical observations were made in preparing compounds **1–4**. First, compound **1**, which is derived from the hydrolysis of flunitrazepam, remains underivatized even though it contained a secondary amino group, apparently because of the steric hindrance and the deactivation effect of the electron withdrawing nitro group in the *para-* position. Second, it was necessary to carry out the derivatization process at room temperature. Heating compound **1** with reagent resulted in demethylation to form the primary amine followed by derivatization to give a derivative equivalent to that of compound **2**. Therefore, under the reported experimental conditions, compound **1** was totally underivatized, compound **2** was a monoheptafluorobutyrate, and compounds **3** and **4** were diheptafluorobutyrates.

The original method used d_5-oxazepam as internal standard. The retention time for the benzophenone heptafluorobutyrate derived from d_5-oxazepam was 4.98 min, and the ions monitored for this internal standard were *m/z* 432 and 263. The method was later modified by using d_3-7-amino-flunitrazepam as internal standard, which resulted in d_3-analog of compound **3**, with ions at *m/z* 516 and 639 being monitored (Fig. 4).

Table 2
Retention Times and Ions Monitored in the GC/MS Analysis of the Benzophenones Derived from the Acid Hydrolysis and Derivatization of Flunitrazepam and Its Metabolites

Benzodiazepines	Benzophenone derivatives	Retention time (min)	Ions monitored[a] (m/z)
Flunitrazepam	1	7.75	<u>274</u>, 211
3-Hydroxy-flunitrazepam	1		
Norflunitrazepam	2	5.79	<u>456</u>, 333
3-Hydroxy-norflunitrazepam	2		
7-Amino-flunitrazepam	3	5.90	<u>513</u>, 636, 423
7-Acetamido-flunitrazepam	3		
7-Amino-3-hydroxy-flunitrazepam	3		
7-Acetamido-3-hydroxy-flunitrazepam	3		
7-Amino-norflunitrazepam	4	5.49	<u>453</u>, 622, 499
7-Acetamido-norflunitrazepam	4		
7-Amino-3-hydroxy-norflunitrazepam	4		
7-Acetamido-3-hydroxy-norflunitrazepam	4		

[a] The quantitation ions are underlined.

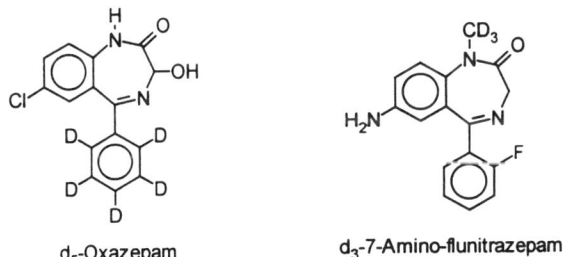

Fig. 4. Structures of d_5-oxazepam and d_3-7-amino-flunitrazepam.

In this procedure, 4 mL of urine sample was spiked with the internal standard, and 1 mL of concentrated hydrochloric acid was added and hydrolysis was carried out at 100°C for 1 h. After extraction with chloroform, the resulting benzophenones were derivatized with heptafluorobutyric anhydride in the presence of 10 µg of 4-pyrolidinopyridine as catalyst at room temperature for 45 min. The heptafluorobutyrate derivatives were chosen because of highest sensitivity and cleanest chromatograms. A capillary DB-5 MS column (25 m × 0.2 mm, 0.33 µm film thickness, J & W Scientific, Folsom, CA) was used with oven temperature programmed as follow: 180°C, held for 0.5 min, then to 260°C at 20°C/min, where it was held for 1.0 min, then to 280°C at 30°C/min and held for 3 min. The retention time and ions for each analyte are listed in Table 2. The LOD and LOQ were 1 ng/mL of each for benzophenone derivatives **3** and **4**. The LOD and LOQ for **1** and **2** were 10 and 25 ng/mL, respectively. The curves were linear up to at least 300 ng/mL. The method was used to determine the concentration of flunitrazepam and its metabolites in urine specimens collected from clinical subjects administered 1-, 2-, and 4-mg doses of flunitrazepam. The results showed that 7-amino-flunitrazepam and 7-aminonorflunitrazepam are the predominant metabolites in urine. The method can detect the presence of flunitrazepam metabolites for at least 72-h post ingestion of a single 1-mg dose.

With some minor modifications, the method was used for analysis of whole blood and serum samples *(50)*. Thus, 1 mL of blood sample spiked with d_3-7-amino-flunitrazepam and d_7-flunitrazepam as internal standards was diluted with 3 mL of HPLC-grade water and the mixture was then analyzed in the same way as discussed for urine samples. The LODs for 7-amino-flunitrazepam, 7-amino-norflunitrazepam, flunitrazepam, and norflunitrazepam were 1, 1, 5, and 5 ng/mL, respectively.

Although this method is sensitive, each of the hydrolysis products actually represent the total amount of the different metabolites that share the same basic skeleton. For example, the concentration of compound **3** is actually the sum of the concentrations of 7-amino-flunitrazepam, 7-amino-3-hydroxy-flunitrazepam, and/or 7-amino-3-hydroxy-flunitrazepam glucuronide conjugate and the corresponding 7-acetamido derivatives. It does not permit the identification of the specific metabolites that are present in urine.

An alternative GC/MS method developed *(10)* by the same group involved enzyme hydrolysis with glucuronidase, liquid–liquid extraction with chloroform–isopropanol (9:1, v/v), and derivatization. Six analytes were divided into two groups: group I contains norflunitrazepam, flunitrazepam, 7-amino-flunitrazepam, 3-hydroxy-flunitrazepam as trimethylsilyl (TMS) derivatives with d_5-oxazepam as internal standard; group II contains 3-hydroxy-norflunitrazepam and 7-amino-3-hydroxy-flunitrazepam as tertiarybutyldimethylsilyl (TBDMS) derivatives with d_5-oxazepam as internal standard. The reported LOD for the major metabolite, 7-aminoflunitrazepam, was 2 ng/mL. This procedure represents one of the early efforts in developing GC/MS methods for identification and analysis of flunitrazepam and its metabolites in urine. Although the procedure seems lengthy, the fact is that routine analysis should be only targeted at 7-amino-flunitrazepam and 7-amino-norflunitrazepam which are the main urinary metabolites, and therefore it is a valuable method due to its sensitivity and low cost.

A recent study reported *(43)* the detection of flunitrazepam and two metabolites in urine by SPE extraction and GC/MS or GC/MS/MS analysis. The drugs were analyzed underivatized. The extraction recoveries by using Bond Elute Certify® ranged from ~80% for flunitrazepam, to 93–100% for 7-amino-flunitrazepam, and 82–100% for norflunitrazepam. The study showed that the enzyme hydrolysis had no effect on the concentrations of 7-amino-flunitrazepam, the major metabolite excreted in urine. Therefore the authors concluded that the enzyme hydrolysis step is unnecessary. Nevertheless, specific data on limit of detection was not reported, although it was stated that GC/MS/MS method was 17-fold more sensitive than regular GC/MS for 7-amino-flunitrazepam based on signal-to-noise ratio.

Elian *(51)* reported a procedure for determination of low levels of flunitrazepam, 7-amino-flunitrazepam, and norflunitrazepam in blood or blood stain by GC/MS using a dual-derivatization procedure. After spiking with the internal standards, d_7-flunitrazepam, d_7-7-amino-flunitrazepam, and d_4-norflunitrazepam, 1 mL of blood sample was diluted with 4 mL of deionized water and 0.2 mL of 100 mM acetic acid and extracted with mixed-mode SPE cartridge (Clean Screen®), which gave recoveries of >90% for each drug. The samples were subsequently derivatized with pentafluoropropionic anhydride (PFPA) first followed by *N-tert*-butyldimethylsilyl-trifluoroacetamide (MTBSTFA) with 1% TBDMSCl. The first step of derivatization with PFPA converts only the primary amino group of 7-amino-flunitrazepam to a pentafluoropropionate. With addition of MTBSTFA with 1% TBDMSCl, norflunitrazepam was converted to its TBDMS derivative, and 7-amino-flunitrazepam is derivatized for the second time. However, flunitrazepam remained underivatized by either reagent. The analytes were separated on an HP-1 column coated with 100% polydimethylsiloxane. As a result, the peak shape and detection sensitivity were largely improved. The limit of detection was 1 ng/mL for each analyte. Table 3 shows some of the parameters for this method.

Two groups recently reported the analysis of flunitrazepam and 7-amino-flunitrazepam in human hair by GC/MS/NCI (negative chemical ionization). The first report *(52)* published in 1997 used d_5-diazepam as internal standard and liquid–liquid extraction with diethyl ether–chloroform (80:20, v/v), after 50 mg of hair was appropriately washed, pulverized, and incubated in 1 mL of phosphate buffer for 2 h at 40°C. The extraction recoveries were 90% for flunitrazepam and 45% for 7-amino-flunitrazepam. After derivatization with heptafluorobutyric anhydride (HFBA) to convert 7-amino-flunitrazepam to heptafluorobutyrate (flunitrazepam was not derivatized), the sample was analyzed using an HP-5 MS capillary column. The limit of detection for flunitrazepam and 7-amino-flunitrazepam was 15 and 3 pg/mg, respectively. The other study

Table 3
Ions, Retention Times, and LODs for Each Analyte by GC/MS Analysis

Compounds	Derivatives	Retention time (min)	Ions monitored	LOD (ng/mL)
Flunitrazepam	Underivatized	7.20	<u>285</u>, 286, 312	1
d$_7$-Flunitrazepam	Underivatized	7.18	<u>292</u>, 293, 318	—
7-Amino-flunitrazepam	PFPA and TBDMS	7.80	<u>486</u>, 487, 246	1
d$_7$-7-Amino-flunitrazepam	PFPA and TBDMS	7.79	<u>493</u>, 494, 340	—
Norflunitrazepam	TBDMS	7.76	<u>356</u>, 357, 310	1
d$_4$-Norflunitrazepam	TBDMS	7.75	<u>360</u>, 361, 314	—

(15) published in 1999 was a modification of the first one in two aspects: use of SPE and deuterated analogs of the analytes (d$_7$-flunitrazepam and d$_7$-7-amino-flunitrazepam) as internal standards. In this procedure, 50 mg of hair was washed with methanol and then digested with 0.1 *N* hydrochloric acid at 55°C overnight. After addition of 1.93 *M* acetic acid, the aqueous digest solution was combined with the methanol wash and passed through a preconditioned mixed-mode SPE column (Isolute® HCX from Lakewood, CO). It was washed with water, 0.1 *N* HCl, and methanol. The sample was eluted with methylene chloride–isopropanol–ammonia (78:20:2) and the extracts were derivatized as HFBA. A 30 m × 250 µm × 0.25 µm HP-5 MS column with GC temperature pro-grammed at 60°C for 1 min, then increased to 310°C at 30°C/min for 6 min. Under these conditions, all compounds were separated within 9–11 min. The ions monitored were *m/z* 313 for flunitrazepam and *m/z* 320 for d$_7$-flunitrazepam; *m/z* 459 for 7-amino-flunitrazepam and *m/z* 466 for d$_7$-7-amino-flunitrazepam. The method was very sensitive with a limit of detection determined to be 1.5 pg/mg and 0.2 pg/mg for flunitrazepam and 7-amino-flunitrazepam, respectively; and the limit of quantitation was 2.5 pg/mg and 0.5 pg/mg for flunitrazepam and 7-amino-flunitrazepam, respectively. Clearly, the enhanced sensitivity as compared to the previous method was attributable to cleaner extracts and the use of deuterated analogs of analytes.

3. Conclusion

The sensitivity and selectivity of the analytical methods used for the determination of flunitrazepam and its metabolites in biological specimens have seen a dramatic improvement over the last decade. This is a direct reflection on the improvement of the tools currently available to forensic toxicologists: from liquid–liquid extraction to solid-phase extraction to immunoaffinity extraction, from HPLC/UV to HPLC/APCI/MS/MS, and from GC/ECD to GC/MS/MS. Although most forensic laboratories still rely heavily on GC/MS, LC/MS has found its niche in forensic applications. In fact, it has become more and more widely used, possibly owing to the reduced cost of equipment in recent years.

This chapter provides a wide range of methods and technologies to assist forensic toxicologists in solving analytical problems involving abuse of flunitrazepam.

References

1. Sternbach, L. H., Fryer, R. I., Keller, O., Metlesics, W., Sach, G., and Steiger, N. (1963) Quinazolines and 1,4-benzodiazepines. X. Nitro-substituted 5-phenyl-1,4-benzodiazepine derivatives. *J. Med. Chem.* **6,** 261.
2. Mattila, M. A. K. and Larni, H. M. (1980) Flunitrazepam: a review of its pharmacological properties and therapeutic use. *Drugs* **20,** 353–374.
3. Baselt, R. C. and Cravey, R. H. (1995) in *Disposition of Toxic Drugs and Chemicals in Man*, 4th edit. Chemical Toxicology Institute, Foster City, CA, pp. 325–327.
4. Flunitrazepam. DEA highlights-1995 http://www.usdoj.gov./dea/pubs/rohypnol/rohypnol.html.
5. Woods, J. H. and Winger, G. (1997) Abuse liability of flunitrazepam. *J. Clin. Psychopharmacol.* **17,** 1S.
6. Calhoun, S. H., Wesson, D. R., Galloway, G. P., and Smith, D. E. (1996) Abuse of flunitrazepam (Rohypnol) and benzodiazepines in Austin and South Texas. *J. Psychoactive Drugs* **28,** 183–189.
7. National Coalition Against Sexual Assault Newsletter (1977) New color-releasing formulation of Rohypnol announced at National NCASA meeting. Cleveland, OH.
8. Saum, C. A. and Inciardi, J. A. (1997) Rohypnol misuse in the United States. *Subst. Use Misuse* **32,** 723.
9. Wendt, G. (1976) Schicksal des hypnotikums Flunitrazepam im menschlichen Organismus, in *Bisherige Erfahrungen mit Rohypnol (Flunitrazepam) in der Anasthesiologie und Intensivtherapie* (Huegin, W., Hossli, G., and Gemperle, M., eds.), Hoffmann-La Roche, Basel, Switzerland, pp. 27–38.
10. Salamone, S. J., Honasoge, S., Brenner, C., McNally, A. J., Passarelli, J., Goc-Szkutnicka, K., et al. (1997) Flunitrazepam excretion patterns using the Abuscreen OnTrack and OnLine Immunoassays: comparison with GC-MS. *J. Analyt. Toxicol.* **21,** 341–345.
11. Dixon, R. (1981) Specific radioimmunoassay for flunitrazepam. *J. Pharmaceut. Sci.* **70,** 230–231.
12. Bruhwyler, J. and Hassoun, A. (1992) The use of radioreceptor assays for the determination of benzodiapines in biological samples: a review. *J. Analyt. Toxicol.* **16,** 244–252.

13. Beck, C., Lafolie, P., Hjemdahl, P., Borg, S., Odelius, G., and Wirbing, P. (1992) Detection of benzodiazepine intake in therapeutic doses by immunoanalysis of urine: two techniques evaluated and modified for improved performance. *Clin. Chem.* **38,** 271–275.
14. Morland, H. and Smith-Kielland, A. (1997) Urine screening for flunitrazepam: applicability of Emit® immunoassay. *Clin. Chem.* **43,** 1245–1246.
15. Negrusz, A., Moore, C., Deitermann, D., Lewis, D., Kaleciak, K., Kronstrand, R., et al. (1999) Highly sensitive micro-plate enzyme immunoassay screening and NCI-GC-MS confirmation of flunitrazepam and its major metabolite 7-aminoflunitrzpam in hair. *J. Analyt. Toxicol.* **23,** 429–435.
16. Walshe, K., Barrett, A. M., Kavanagh, P. V., McNamara, S. M., Moran, C., and Shattock, A. G. (2000) A sensitive immunoassay for flunitrazepam and metabolites. *J. Analyt. Toxicol.* **24,** 296–299.
17. Haefelfinger, P. (1975) Determination of nanogram amounts of primary aromatic amines and nitro compounds in blood and plasma. *J. Chromatogr.* **111,** 323–329.
18. Battista, H. J. (1979) Detection of benzodiazepines in forensic chemistry. *Beitr. Gerichtl. Med.* **37,** 5–28.
19. De Bruyne, M. M. A., Sinnema, A., and Verweij, A. M. A. (1984) Hydrolysis of clonazepam, flunitrazepam and nitrazepam by hydrochloric acid identification of some additional products. *Forensic Sci. Int.* **24,** 125–135.
20. Van Rooij, H. H., Fakiera, A., and Verrijk, R. (1985) Identification of flunitrazepam and its metabolites in urine sample. *Analyt. Chim. Acta.* **170,** 153–158.
21. Haefelfinger, P. (1979) Determination of the 7-amino metabolites of the 7-nitrobenzodiazepines in human plasma by thin layer chromatography. *J. High Res. Chromatogr. Chromatogr. Commun.* **2,** 39–42.
22. Faber, D. B., Kok, R. M., and Rempt-van Dijk, E. M. (1977) Quantitative gas chromatographic analysis of flunitrazepam in human serum with electron-capture detection. *J. Chromatogr.* **133,** 319–326.
23. Cano, J. P., Guintrand, J., Aubert, C., and Aubert, C. (1977) Determination of flunitrazepam, desmethylflunitrazepam and clonazepam in plasma by gas chromatography with an internal standard. *Arzneim-Forsch.* **27,** 338–342.
24. De Silva, J. A. F., Puglisi, C. V., and Munno, N. (1974) Determination of clonazepam and flunitrazepam in blood by EC-GLC. *J. Pharmaceut. Sci.* **68,** 520–526.
25. Jochemsen, R. and Breimer, D. D. (1982) Assay of flunitrazepam, tempazepam and desalkylflunitrazepam in plasma by capillary GC with ECD. *J. Chromatogr.* **227,** 199–206.
26. Lillsunde, P. and Seppala, T. (1990) Simultaneous screening and quantitative analysis of benzodiazepines by dual-channel gas chromatography using electron-capture and nitrogen-phosphorus detection. *J. Chromatogr.* **533,** 97–110.
27. Maurer, H. and Pfleger, K. (1981) Determination of 1,4- and 1,5-benzodiazepines in urine using a computerized gas chromatographic-mass spectrometric technique. *J. Chromatogr.* **222,** 409–419.
28. Drouet-Coassolo, C., Aubert, C., Coassolo, P., and Cano, J. P. (1989) Capillary gas chromatographic mass spectrometric method for the identification and quantifica-

tion of some benzodiazepines and their unconjugated metabolites in plasma. *J. Chromatogr.* **487,** 295–311.
29. Vree, T. B., Linselbink, B., Van der Klein, E., and Nijhus, G. M. M. (1977) Determination of flunitrazepam in body fluids by means of high performance liquid chromatography. *J. Chromatogr.* **143,** 530–534.
30. Sumirtapura, Y. C., Aubert, C., Coassolo, P., and Cano, P. J. (1982) Determination of 7-aminoflunitrazepam (Ro 20-1815) and 7-amino-desmethylflunitrazepam (Ro 5-4650) in plasma by high performance liquid chromatography and fluorescence detection. *J. Chromatogr.* **232,** 111–118.
31. Weijers-Everhard, J. P., Wijker, J., Verrijk, R., Van Rooij, H., and Soudijn, W. (1986) Improved quantitative method for establishing flunitrazepam abuse using urine sample and column liquid chromatography with flurometric detection. *J. Chromatogr.* **374,** 339–346.
32. West, A., Köhler-Schmidt, H., Baudner, S., and Blaschke, G. (1995) A specific immunoassay for the detection of flunitrazepam. *Int. J. Legal. Med.* **108,** 105–109.
33. Boukhabza, A., Lugnier, A. A. J., Kintz, P., and Mangin, P. (1991) Simultaneous HPLC analysis of the hypnotic benzodiazepines nitrazepam, estazolam, flunitrazepam, and triazolam in plasma. *J. Analyt. Toxicol.* **15,** 319–322.
34. Cornelissen, P. J. and Beijersbergen van Henegouwen, G. M. (1979) Photochemical decomposition of 1,4-benzodiazepines. Nitrazepam. *Photochem. Photobiol.* **30,** 337–341.
35. Berthault, F., Kintz, P., and Mangin, P. (1996) Simultaneous high-performance liquid chromatographic analysis of flunitrazepam and four metabolites in serum. *J. Chromatogr.* **685,** 383–387.
36. Darius, J. and Banditt, P. (2000) Validated method for the therapeutic drug monitoring of flunitrazepam in human serum using liquid chromatography-atmospheric pressure chemical ionization tandem mass spectrometry with an ion trap detector. *J. Chromatogr.* **738,** 437–441.
37. Benhamou-Batut, F., Demotes-Mainard, F., Labat, L., Vincon, G., and Bannwarth, B. (1994) Determination of flunitrazepam in plasma by liquid chromatography. *J. Pharmaceut. Biomed. Anal.* **12,** 931–936.
38. McIntyre, I. M., Syrjanen, M. L., Crump, K., Horomidis, S., and Peace, A. W. (1993) Simultaneous HPLC gradient analysis of 15 benzodiazepines and selected metabolites in postmortem blood. *J. Analyt. Toxicol.* **17,** 202–207.
39. Chen, X. H., Franke, J. P., van Veen, J., Wijsbeek, J., and de Zeeuw, R. A. (1990) Solid-phase extraction for the screening of acidic, neutral and basic drugs in plasma using a single-column procedure on Bond Elut Certify. *J. Chromatogr.* **529,** 161–166.
40. Moore, C. M. (1990) Solid phase cation exchange extraction of basic drugs from urine of racing greyhounds. *J. Forensic Sci. Soc.* **30,** 123–129.
41. He, W. and Parissis, N. (1997) Simultaneous determination of flunitrazepam and its metabolites in plasma and urine by HPLC/DAD after solid phase extraction. *J. Pharmaceut. Biomed. Anal.* **16,** 707–715.
42. Reynolds, J. E. F. ed. (1993) Martindale, *The Extra Pharmacopoeia,* 30th edit. Pharmaceutical Press, London, pp. 595.

43. Nguyen, N. and Nau, D. R. (2000) Rapid method for the solid-phase extraction and GC-MS analysis of flunitrazepam and its major metabolites in urine. *J. Analyt. Toxicol.* **24,** 37–45.
44. Guichard, J., Panteix, G., Dubost, J., Baltassat, P., and Roche, C. (1993) Simultaneous high-performance liquid chromatographic assay of droperidol and flunitrazepam in human plasma. Application to haemodilution blood samples collected during clinical anaesthesia. *J. Chromatogr.* **612,** 269–275.
45. Bogusz, M. J., Maier, R.-D., Krüger, K.-D., and Früchtnicht, W. (1998) Determination of flunitrazepam and its metabolites in blood by high-performance liquid chromatography-atmospheric pressure chemical ionization mass spectrometry. *J. Chromatogr.* **713,** 361–369.
46. Deinl, I., Mahr, G., and von Meyer, L. (1998) Determination of flunitrazepam and its main metabolites in serum and urine by HPLC after mixed-mode solid-phase extraction. *J. Analyt. Toxicol.* **22,** 197–202.
47. Deinl, I., Angermaier, L., Franzelius, C., and Machbert, G. (1997) Simple high-performance liquid chromatographic column-switching technique for the on-line immunoaffinity extraction and analysis of flunitrazepam and its main metabolites in urine. *J. Chromatogr.* **704,** 251–258.
48. Deinl, I., Franzelius, C., Angermaier, L., Mahr, C., and Machbert, G. (1999) On-line immunoaffinity extraction and HPLC analysis of flunitrazepam and its main metabolites in serum. *J. Analyt. Toxicol.* **23,** 598–602.
49. ElSohly, M. A., Feng, S., Salamone, S. J., and Wu, R. (1997) A sensitive procedure for the analysis of flunitrazepam and its metabolites in urine. *J. Analyt. Toxicol.* **21,** 335–340.
50. ElSohly, M. A., Feng, S., Salamone, S. J., and Brenneisen, R. (1999) GC–MS determination of flunitrazepam and its major metabolites in whole blood and plasma. *J. Analyt. Toxicol.* **23,** 486–489.
51. Elian, A. A. (1999) Detection of low levels of flunitrazepam and its metabolites in blood and bloodstains. *Forensic Sci. Int.* **101,** 107–111 (1999).
52. Cirimele, V., Kintz, P., Staub, C., and Mangin, P. (1997) Testing human hair for flunitrazepam and 7-amino-flunitrazepam by GC/MS-NCI. *Forensic Sci. Int.* **84,** 189–200.

Chapter 4

Analysis of Selected Low-Dose Benzodiazepines by Mass Spectrometry

Dennis J. Crouch and Matthew H. Slawson

1. INTRODUCTION

The benzodiazepines discussed in this chapter are alprazolam, lorazepam, midazolam, and triazolam. They are all prescription medications that are used as anti-anxiety agents, preoperative medications, or as sedative–hypnotics *(1)*. All are prescribed in very low doses (because of their potency), rapidly metabolized, and have short plasma half-lives (Table 1). Generally, they are biotransformed to hydroxylated metabolites and are excreted in the urine as glucuronide conjugates. Because the recommended therapeutic doses of alprazolam, lorazepam, midazolam, and triazolam may be 1 mg or less and the drugs are rapidly metabolized, plasma concentrations of the parent drugs and their metabolites are in nanogram per milliliter concentrations. Therefore, the detection and quantification of alprazolam, lorazepam, midazolam, triazolam, and their respective metabolites present a significant challenge to the analytical laboratory.

Commercial laboratory-based and on-site benzodiazepine immunoassay test kits are designed primarily to detect urinary metabolites of diazepam. Therefore, these tests usually have limited utility for the detection of the potent benzodiazepines discussed in this chapter. The limitations of these commercial immunoassay tests for the detection of alprazolam, lorazepam, midazolam, triazolam, and their urinary metabolites are discussed in other sections of this book and

From: *Forensic Science: Benzodiazepines and GHB: Detection and Pharmacology*
Edited by: S. J. Salamone © Humana Press Inc., Totowa, NJ

Table 1
Pharmacokinetic Data:
Alprazolam, Lorazepam, Midazolam, and Triazolam

Drug	$t_{1/2}$ (h)	Therapeutic uses	Therapeutic concentrations	Major metabolite(s)
Alprazolam	10–15	Antianxiety, panic disorder	20–40 ng/mL	α-Hydroxyalprazolam and 4-hydroxyalprazolam
Lorazepam	10–25	Antianxiety, sedative, preoperative	150–250 ng/mL	Conjugated lorazepam
Midazolam	1.3–2.5	Preoperative sedative	30–70 ng/mL	1-Hydroxymidazolam and 4-hydroxymidazolam
Triazolam	1.5–5.5	Hypnotic	3–5 ng/mL	α-Hydroxytriazolam and 4-hydroxytriazolam

Data from ref. *1*.

reviewed in the literature *(2)*. Detection of alprazolam, lorazepam, and triazolam by laboratory-based immunoassays has been reported *(3)*. However, this method required extraction of the blood and only alprazolam was consistently detected.

Numerous gas chromatographic (GC) methods have been published for the analysis of alprazolam, lorazepam, midazolam, and triazolam and their metabolites from various biological specimens. The most effective GC methods used electron capture detection (ECD) or mass spectrometry (MS) detection. ECD was needed to obtain the sensitivity and specificity required to detect and quantify the drugs and metabolites discussed in this chapter, especially when analyzing blood and plasma samples *(2)*. The most specific GC methods have used MS detection. These methods are the focus of this chapter.

The GC/MS methods for the analysis of alprazolam, lorazepam, midazolam, triazolam, and their metabolites in urine follow a similar outline. The urine sample is treated by enzymatic hydrolysis to cleave metabolite–glucuronide bonds. The drugs and metabolites are extracted into an organic solvent. The solvent is evaporated and the metabolites derivatized prior to analysis using capillary column GC/MS with electron ionization (EI) mass spectrometry.

The detection and quantification of alprazolam, lorazepam, midazolam, triazolam, and their metabolites in specimens other than urine may be problematic using EI GC/MS. EI GC/MS analyses are particularly problematic following therapeutic doses of the drugs because expected drug and metabolite concentrations are quite low. Therefore, many of the methods presented in this chapter for the analysis of these drugs and their metabolites in blood, plasma, and tissues use alternate techniques and more sophisticated MS techniques such as chemical ionization and MS/MS. A major advantage of high-performance liquid chromatography (HPLC) for the analysis of benzodiazepine drugs is that no derivatization of the metabolites is required. Further, improved chromatographic peak shape may also be observed for the parent drugs. The development of new ionization techniques has made HPLC/MS and HPLC/MS/MS extremely effective analytical tools for the analysis of of alprazolam, lorazepam, midazolam, and triazolam and their respective metabolites. These techniques are discussed in the following sections.

2. ALPRAZOLAM

2.1. Background

Alprazolam is a 1,4-triazolo analog of the 1,4-benzodiazepines (Fig. 1). In the United States, alprazolam is available in tablet form in doses of 0.25, 0.5, 1.0, and 2.0 mg *(4)*. It is prescribed in doses up to 4.0 mg/day and used primarily as an anxiolytic *(4)*. Alprazolam is one of the most frequently reported

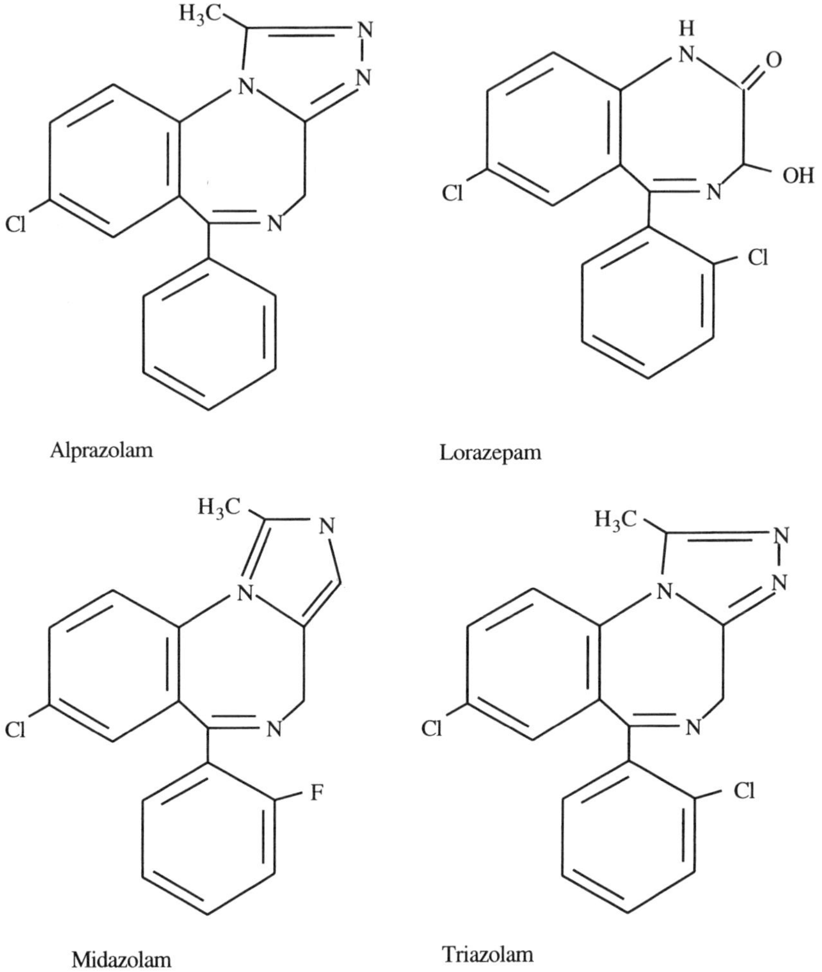

Alprazolam

Lorazepam

Midazolam

Triazolam

Fig. 1. Chemical structure of the four benzodiazepines discussed in this chapter. They are usually prescribed in low doses as anxiety agents, preoperative medications, or as sedative-hypnotics. The dosage and rapid metabolization of these compounds present a significant challenge to the analytical laboratory because their plasma concentrations are usually in the nanogram per milliliter range.

prescription drugs in emergency departments (5). However, the toxicity of alprazolam is relatively low, and it is generally reported in emergency toxicology cases in combination with other drugs. Following oral doses, alprazolam is rapidly absorbed and peak plasma concentrations are reached within 1–2 h after administration (6,7). After a single 1-mg dose of alprazolam was administered to 10 subjects, mean peak plasma concentrations were 11.5 ng/mL *(8)*. Pharmacokinetic studies have demonstrated that there is a relatively predictable relationship between dose and plasma concentration. For each milligram of alprazolam administered, the resulting plasma concentration is increased by approx 10–20 ng/mL *(6–8)*. Alprazolam is extensively metabolized and its principal metabolites are α-hydroxyalprazolam, a benzophenone, and 4-hydroxyalprazolam *(6,7,9,10)*. However, only the α-hydroxyalprazolam metabolite appears to have pharmacological activity *(6,7,9,10)*. Pharmacokinetic studies indicate that the α- and 4-hydroxy metabolites of alprazolam can be detected in plasma, but that concentrations of these metabolites (in unconjugated form) are considerably lower (<10%) than those of the parent drug *(6–10)*. After a single 1-mg dose of alprazolam, mean peak plasma α-hydroxyalprazolam concentrations were 0.18 ng/mL *(8)*. Alprazolam is primarily eliminated in the urine as metabolites, with the parent drug representing up to 20% of the urinary products *(9)*.

As stated in the introduction, commercial laboratory-based and on-site immunoassay tests have been developed primarily to detect urinary metabolites of diazepam. Therefore, these tests have limited utility for the detection of alprazolam and its metabolites in urine or other biological specimens. Their value is also limited because plasma and urinary concentrations of alprazolam and its metabolites are much less than those of diazepam and its metabolites. Numerous GC methods have been reported for the analysis of alprazolam and its metabolites *(11,12)*. The most effective methods used ECD *(11–13)*. However, improved specificity for the analysis of alprazolam and α-hydroxyalprazolam has been obtained through the use of capillary column GC/MS with EI *(14–16)*. Most urinary methods utilized enzymatic hydrolysis, and trimethylsilyl derivatives of the polar alprazolam metabolites were formed prior to instrumental analysis *(15,16)*. Several authors have demonstrated that negative ion chemical ionization (NICI) GC/MS is even more selective and sensitive than conventional EI for the analysis of alprazolam and its metabolites *(9,17,18)*. Fitzgerald et al. *(17)* reported that for the analysis of α-hydroxyalprazolam, NICI was 500 times more sensitive than EI and 200 times more sensitive than positive ion chemical ionization (PICI). Outlined in the following section is an NICI GC/MS method for the analysis of alprazolam and α-hydroxyalprazolam in plasma *(9)*.

2.2. Method 1

2.2.1. Extraction

Calibration curves for alprazolam and α-hydroxyalprazolam were prepared by fortifying plasma at 0, 0.25, 0.50, 1.0, 2.5, 5.0, 7.5, 10.0, 25.0, and

50.0 ng/mL. Ten nanograms of triazolam-d_4 and 5 ng of α-hydroxyalprazolam-d_5 were added as internal standards. (The authors explained that they were unable to obtain significantly pure deuterium-labeled alprazolam.) The tubes were mixed, allowed to equilibrate at ambient temperature for at least 30 min, made basic by adding 1 mL of saturated sodium borate buffer (pH 9), and the analytes were extracted into 7 mL of toluene–methylene chloride (7:3). The organic phase was transferred to an evaporation tube and evaporated under a stream of air. The residues were reconstituted in 25 µL of ethyl acetate followed by 25 µL of BSTFA + 1% TMCS (*N,O-bis*-[trimethylsilyl]trifluoroacetamide–1% trimethylchlorosilane) and then heated at 80°C for at least 30 min to derivatize the α-hydroxyalprazolam. The tubes were allowed to cool to room temperature and the liquid transferred to autosampler vials for analysis.

2.2.2. GC/MS Conditions

Methane was used as the NICI regent gas. The MS was programmed to acquire selection ion monitoring (SIM) data for the following *m/z*: alprazolam, 308; triazolam-d_4, 310; α-hydroxyalprazolam, 396; and α-hydroxyalprazolam-d_5, 401. A 15-m capillary column with a 0.25 mm internal diameter (i.d.), 0.25 µm film thickness was used with hydrogen as the carrier gas. The initial GC temperature of 190°C was held for 1 min, then programmed to 320°C at the rate of 20°/min. A representative chromatogram is shown in Fig. 2.

2.2.3. Method Performance

The extraction recoveries for alprazolam and α-hydroxyalprazolam were 108.0% and 75.5%, respectively at 1 ng/mL and 100.8% and 99.4%, respectively at 50 ng/mL. The method was linear for both alprazolam and α-hydroxyalprazolam from 0.25 to 50 ng/mL. The accuracy and precision of the method were experimentally determined at 0.5, 5.0, and 50 ng/mL. For alprazolam, the intraassay precision was approx 16% coefficient of variation (CV) at 0.5 ng/mL, <6% CV at 5.0 ng/mL, and <5% CV at 50 ng/mL. The interassay precision was approx 16% CV at 0.5 ng/mL, approx 15% CV at 5.0 ng/mL, and <10% CV at 50 ng/mL. For α-hydroxyalprazolam, the intraassay precision was approx 16% CV at 0.5 ng/mL, <7% CV at 5.0 ng/mL, and <5% CV at 50 ng/mL. The interassay precision was <6% CV at 0.5 ng/mL, <9% CV at 5.0 ng/mL, and 9% CV at 50 ng/mL. The intraassay accuracy for alprazolam was within 4.4% of target at 0.5 ng/mL, 15% at 5.0 ng/mL, and approx 1% at 50 ng/mL. The interassay accuracy for alprazolam was within 6% of target at 0.5 ng/mL, 7% at 5.0 ng/mL, and approx 1% at 50 ng/mL. The intraassay accuracy for α-hydroxyalprazolam was within 3.0% of target at 0.5 ng/mL, approx 4% at 5.0 ng/mL, and within 10% at 50 ng/mL. The interassay accuracy for α-hydroxy-

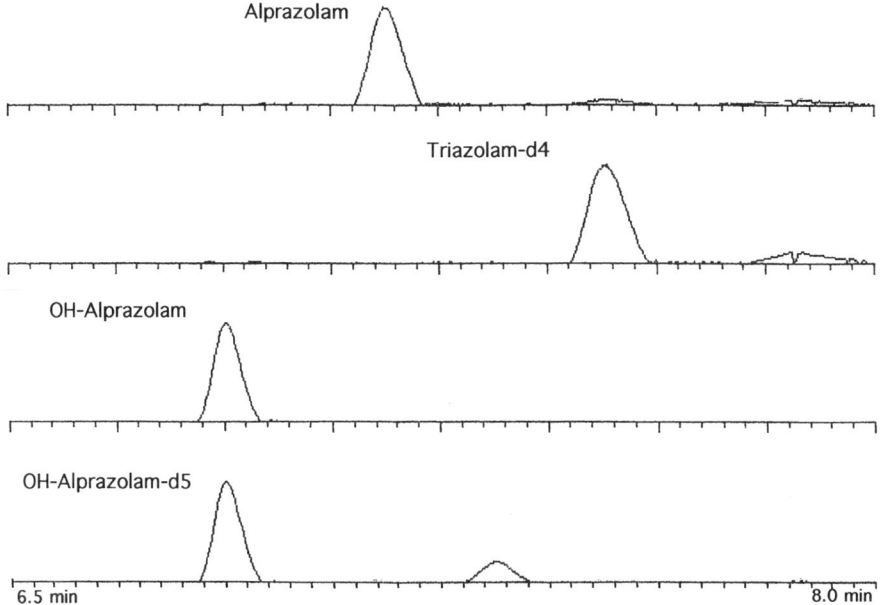

Fig. 2. Sample chromatogram from NICI GC/MS analysis of 0.05 ng/mL α-hydroxyalprazolam and alprazolam and their deuterated internal standards.

alprazolam was within 9% of target at 0.5 ng/mL, 4% at 5.0 ng/mL, and approximately 1% at 50 ng/mL.

2.3. Method 2

A major disadvantage of GC methods for the analysis of alprazolam, 4-hydroxyalprazolam, and α-hydroxyalprazolam is the need to derivatize the metabolites to obtain Gaussian chromatographic peaks. However, α-hydroxyalprazolam and 4-hydroxyalprazolam can be analyzed by HPLC without derivatization *(19–21)*. McIntyre et al. *(20),* used gradient HPLC to analyze 15 different benzodiazepines including alprazolam in whole blood samples. Lambert et al. *(21)* demonstrated that HPLC could be used to analyze blood, urine, stomach contents, and tissue samples for alprazolam and a variety of other benzodiazepines and their metabolites. Recent developments in HPLC/MS, such as atmospheric pressure ionization techniques and the availability of lower cost instruments, have made HPLC/MS and HPLC/MS/MS the analysis techniques of choice for many benzodiazepines. Kleinschnitz et al. *(22)* reported an HPLC/MS/MS method using solid-phase extraction capable of quantifying 2 ng/mL of 1,4-benzodiazepines from serum and urine *(22)*. Crouch et al. *(8)* reported an HPLC/MS/MS using electrospray ionization (ESI) capable of detecting and quantifying 0.05 ng/mL of alprazolam and α-hydroxyalprazolam in human plasma. This method is outlined in the following section (8).

2.3.1. Extraction

The extraction procedure was a modification of that published by Hold et al. (9) and presented in the preceding section (9). Plasma, blood, or urine calibration curves contained the following concentrations of alprazolam and α-hydroxyalprazolam: 0.0, 0.05, 0.10, 0.25, 0.50, 1.0, 2.5, 5.0, 10.0, 25.0, and 50.0 ng/mL. Five nanograms of alprazolam-d_5 and α-hydroxyalprazolam-d_5 were added to each tube. Urine samples were hydrolyzed using β-glucuronidase and incubation. The samples were buffered and extracted as explained earlier. After drying, the residues were reconstituted in 80 μL of HPLC solvent, centrifuged, and the supernatant transferred to autosampler vials.

2.3.2. HPLC/MS/MS Conditions

The analyses were performed with a tandem quadruple mass spectrometer using ESI with positive ion detection. A 150-mm × 2.1-mm i.d. C18 HPLC column was used. The HPLC was operated isocratically at a flow rate of 250 μL/min. The solvent was methanol–water (60:40) containing 0.1% formic acid. A sample chromatogram is shown in Fig. 3. The tube lens, capillary voltages, and MS/MS conditions were optimized for the detection of alprazolam and α-hydroxyalprazolam. Nitrogen was used as the sheath gas and the auxiliary gas. The mass spectrometer was operated in the selected reaction monitoring (SRM) detection mode. The transitions monitored were products of alprazolam (m/z = 309–205), alprazolam-d_5 (m/z = 314–209), α-hydroxyalprazolam (m/z = 325–216), and α-hydroxyalprazolam-d_5 (m/z = 330–221). Product ion spectra of alprazolam and α-hydroxyalprazolam are shown in Fig. 4.

2.3.3. Method Performance

The extraction recoveries for alprazolam at 1, 10, and 50 ng/mL were 88%, 99%, and 85%, respectively. The extraction efficiencies for alprazolam at 1, 10, and 50 ng/mL were 102%, 85%, and 78%, respectively. The method was linear for both alprazolam and α-hydroxyalprazolam from 0.05 to 50 ng/mL. The accuracy and precision of the method were experimentally determined at 2.0, 5.0, and 20 ng/mL. For alprazolam, the intraassay precision was approx <6% CV at 2.0 ng/mL, <4% CV at 5.0 ng/mL, and <5% CV at 50 ng/mL. The interassay precision was approx 12% CV at 2.0 ng/mL, <9% CV at 5.0 ng/mL, and <9% CV at 50 ng/mL. For α-hydroxyalprazolam, the intraassay precision was <9% CV at 2.0 ng/mL, <5% CV at 5.0 ng/mL, and <5% CV at 50 ng/mL.

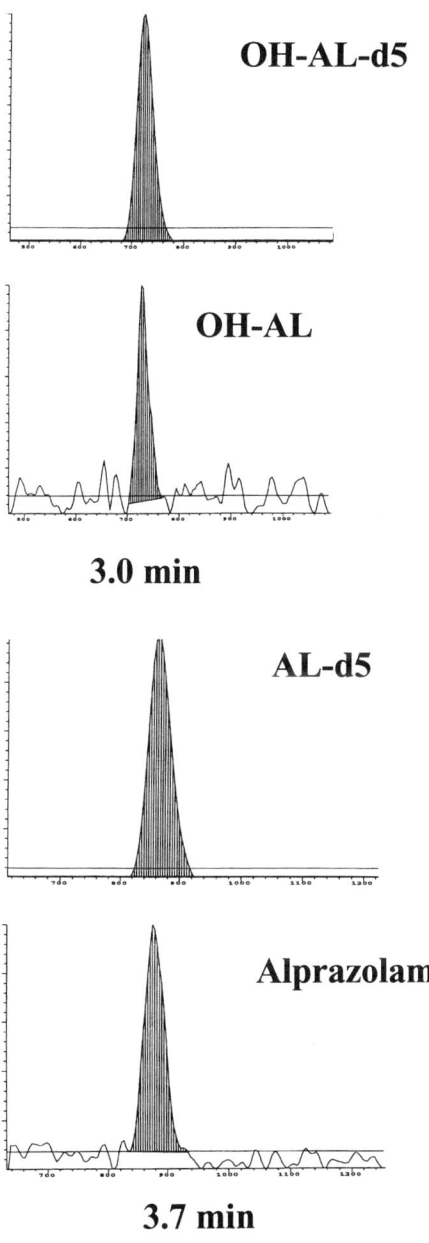

Fig. 3. Sample chromatogram from HPLC/MS/MS analysis of 0.05 ng/mL α-hydroxyalprazolam (OH-AL) and alprazolam and their deuterated internal standards. Reproduced from the *Journal of Analytical Toxicology* by permission of Preston Publications, a division of Preston Industries, Inc.

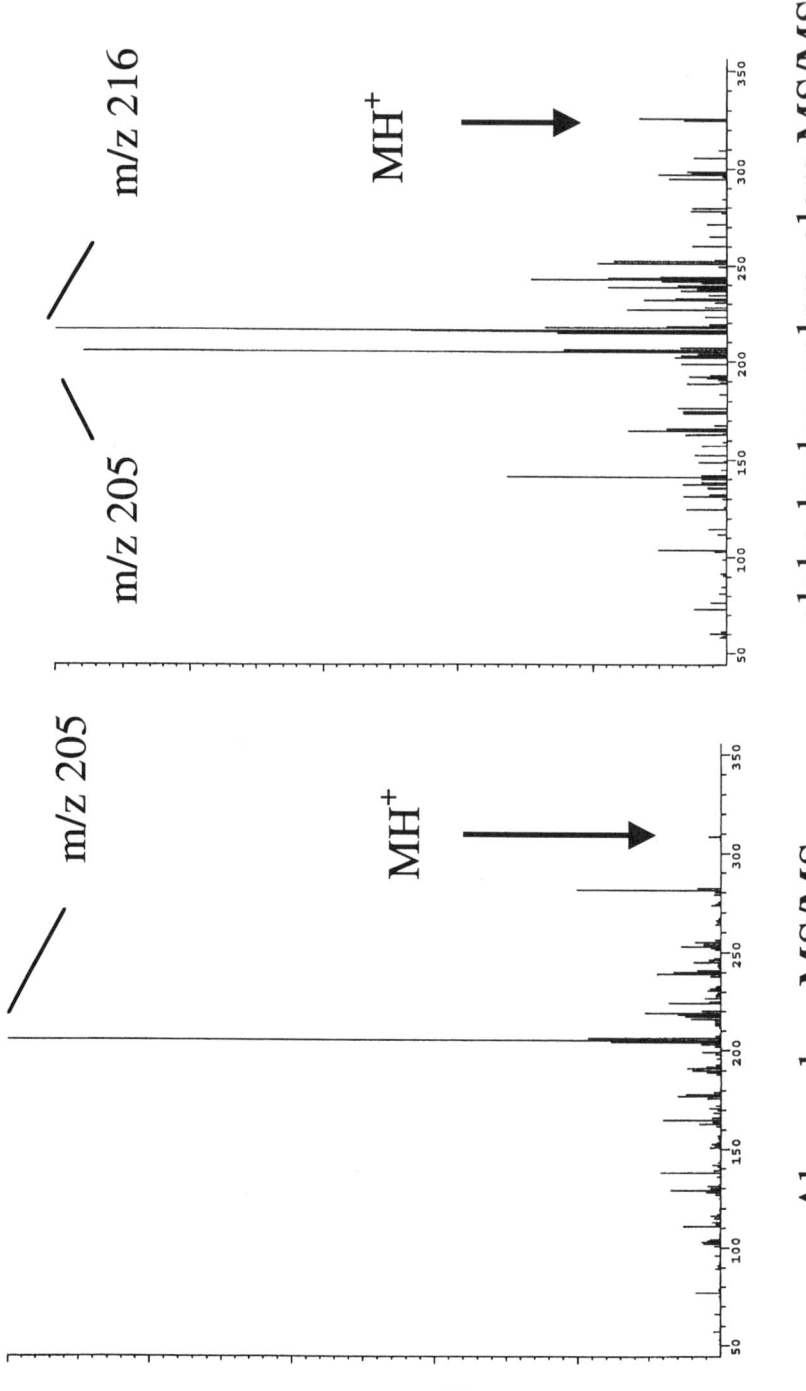

Fig. 4. MS/MS product ion spectra of α-hydroxyalprazolam and alprazolam. Reproduced from the *Journal of Analytical Toxicology* by permission of Preston Publications, a division of Preston Industries, Inc.

The interassay precision was <10% CV at 2.0 ng/mL, <10% CV at 5.0 ng/mL, and <8% CV at 50 ng/mL. The accuracy of the method was calculated by comparing the mean assayed concentration with the target concentration of quality-control samples fortified at 2.0, 10, and 50 ng/mL of alprazolam and α-hydroxy-alprazolam. All mean control concentrations were within ± 6.6% of their target values.

3. MIDAZOLAM

3.1. Background

Midazolam (Versed®) is a fluorinated 1,4-imadazo analog of the 1,4-benzodiazepines (Fig. 1). It has a short half-life (approx 2 h) and is metabolized to pharmacologically active 1-hydroxymidazolam and inactive 4-hydroxymidazolam. Both metabolites undergo phase II glucuronidation and are eliminated primarily in the urine. Midazolam has become a popular adjunct to anesthesia because it is water soluble, and has a rapid onset and short duration of action *(1)*. In the United States, it is available in an injectable form at 1 and 5 mg/mL concentrations in 1-, 2-, 5-, and 10-mL vials *(4)*. It is also available as a syrup primarily for pediatric use *(4)*. After a single 7.5-mg intramuscular (i.m.) injection of midazolam, peak plasma concentrations of 90 ng/mL were observed at 0.5 h *(4)*. A peak plasma concentration of 8 ng/mL of the 1-hydroxy metabolite was observed at 1 h. After oral administration, midazolam is rapidly absorbed and is subjected to first-pass metabolism. In pediatric populations (6 mo–16 yr), the pharmacokinetics of oral midazolam vary considerably. A peak plasma concentration of 28 ng/mL was reported at 0.17 h after a 0.25-mg oral dose, and a mean peak concentration of 191 ± 47 ng/mL was reported at 0.55 ± 0.28 h after a 1-mg oral dose *(4)*. In adults ($n = 10$), average peak plasma concentrations of 69 ng/mL were observed in men at approx 1 h after a 10-mg oral dose and 59 ng/mL in women after the same dose *(23)*.

Midazolam and its metabolites have been analyzed by immunoassay, GC with ECD, nitrogen-selective detection, and mass spectrometry *(15,24–31)*.

3.2. Method 1

3.2.1. Extraction

Martens and Banditt described a method for the determination of midazolam, α-hydroxy, and 4-hydroxymidazolam in human serum utilizing GC/MS *(32)*. One milliliter of serum was fortified with internal standard and 100 μL of 0.1 M NaOH was added. The sample was extracted twice with 2 mL of toluene containing 20 μL of amyl alcohol. After the extraction, the organic layer was collected and evaporated to dryness. The sample extract was derivatized with 50 µL of *N*-methyl-*N*-*t*-butyldimethylsilyl trifluoroacetamide (MTBSTFA) for 30 min at 60°C. Excess derivatizing reagent was removed by evaporation under vacuum and the residue was reconstituted in 50 µL ethyl acetate.

3.2.2. GC/MS Conditions

Chromatographic separation was achieved using a nonpolar capillary column (15 m × 0.25 mm i.d. and 5 µm film thickness) with helium as the carrier gas. The initial column temperature was held at 85°C for 1 min. The temperature was increased at a rate of 30°C per minute to 200°C, then 10°C per minute to 310°C. The final temperature was held for 2 min. The injector and interface temperatures were 300°C. SIM data were collected.

3.2.3. Method Performance

The method had a limit of detection of 0.2 ng/mL for midazolam and 0.1 ng/mL for the metabolites. The authors reported an extraction efficiency recovery of 83–96% for midazolam and its metabolites with acceptable precision and accuracy for all analytes. Methods utilizing liquid chromatography have also been reported *(33–37)*.

3.3. Method 2

Recently methods using HPLC coupled to MS have been published for the analysis of midazolam and its metabolites. Kanazawa et al. *(38)* describe a method utilizing atmospheric pressure chemical ionization (APCI) HPLC/MS for the quantitative analysis of a variety of benzodiazepines including midazolam *(38)*.

3.3.1. Extraction

Drug-fortified canine plasma (200 µL) was extracted using solid-phase extraction as follows: C18 cartridges were pretreated with water, methanol, and 0.1 *M* ammonium acetate; the samples were applied and the cartridges were washed with ammonium acetate; the analytes were eluted with methanol–ammonium acetate (3:1).

3.3.2. HPLC/MS Conditions

Chromatographic separation was achieved at ambient temperature using a 150 mm × 4.6 mm reverse-phase HPLC column. The mobile phase consisted of methanol–0.1 *M* ammonium acetate (3:2). Other analytical details were not provided.

3.3.3. Method Performance

The authors reported sensitivity limits of 10–50 pg of analyte per injection, a dynamic range of 0–500 ng per injection, and a recovery of 96.1% for midazolam. Details of the precision and accuracy of the assay were not given.

3.4. Method 3

A method using ESI HPLC/MS for the detection of midazolam and 1-hydroxymidazolam in human serum was reported by Marquet et al. in 1999 *(39)*.

3.4.1. Extraction

Two-mL aliquots of serum plus internal standard were made basic by adding carbonate buffer, pH 9.5. Samples were extracted with 8 mL of diethyl ether–2-propanol. After extraction, the organic phase was evaporated to dryness under nitrogen. Samples were reconstituted in the mobile phase prior to injection.

3.4.2. HPLC/MS Conditions

Chromatographic separation was achieved using a mobile phase of acetonitrile and 5 mM ammonium formate, pH 3, gradient elution, and a reversed phase HPLC column. The MS was equipped with an ESI source and utilized nitrogen for the curtain and nebulization gases. In-source fragmentation was achieved by optimizing the orifice voltage for each analyte. Positive ions were detected by SIM acquisition. Data from two ions were collected for each analyte. One ion served as the quantitation ion and the other served as a qualifier for qualitative identification.

3.4.3. Method Performance

Recovery of the analytes was reported as >79% at three concentrations. The limit of detection (as defined by a minimum signal-to-noise ratio of 3 to 1) was 0.2 ng/mL for midazolam and 0.5 ng/mL for the metabolite. Intraassay precision was reported as <15% CV ($n = 6$) for all analytes and interassay precision was <20% CV for all analytes through the dynamic range of the assay, with the exception of the limit of detection (LOD) (0.2 ng/mL), which had a 24.7% CV.

3.5. Additional Techniques

Lausecker et al. *(40)* compared methods using capillary zone electrophoresis (CZE) and micro-HPLC using an ESI-MS for the analysis of midazolam and its metabolites. They also compared liquid–liquid extraction and solid-phase extraction for sample preparation prior to analysis. Their conclusions were that CZE/MS/MS combined with a liquid–liquid extraction provided limits of detection superior to the other methods tested. The authors stressed the importance of appropriate sample clean-up prior to analysis to achieve optimal sensitivity and method performance.

4. LORAZEPAM

4.1. Background

Lorazepam (Ativan®) is a 3-hydroxybenzodiazepine that is structurally related to oxazepam and temazepam (Fig. 1). It is available in tablet form (0.5–2 mg) or in solution (2–4 mg/mL) for parenteral administration. It is used clinically as a preanesthetic and for the treatment of anxiety disorders. Lorazepam has a half-life of 9–16 h and is rapidly inactivated by conjugation with glucuronic acid *(41)*. The glucuronide can accumulate and is slowly excreted in the urine (75% of a dose over a 5-d period; *41*). After a single 2-mg oral dose of lorazepam, average plasma concentrations at 2-h were 18 ng/mL and declined to 9 ng/mL by 12 h *(41)*. During chronic daily dosing of 10 mg of lorazepam, steady-state plasma concentrations averaged 181 ng/mL *(42)*. After intramuscular injection of 4 mg of lorazepam, peak plasma concentrations averaged 57 ng/mL at 1.5 h in six subjects *(42)*. This is consistent with the manufacturer's report that a 4-mg i.m. dose of lorazepam resulted in a C_{max} of 48 ng/mL within 3 h *(4)*. A 5-mg intravenous (i.v.) dose of lorazepam resulted in peak plasma concentrations of 140 ng/mL within the first few minutes *(42)*. The manufacturer reports that administration of 4 mg i.v. resulted in initial concentrations of 70 ng/mL *(4)*.

Quantitative analysis of lorazepam in biological specimens has been performed primarily using GC/MS *(17,43–45)*. Fitzgerald et al. *(17)* reported a sensitive method for the analysis of several benzodiazepines, including lorazepam, in urine that used NICI GC/MS *(17)*. The authors compared NICI GC/MS results with PICI and EI GC/MS results.

4.2. Method

4.2.1. Extraction

Urine samples (0.5 mL) were fortified with internal standard and hydrolyzed with β-glucuronidase (5000 U/mL, pH 5) at 70°C for 2 h. Following hydrolysis, the samples were made basic by adding 0.5 mL of saturated borate buffer and extracted with 2 mL of toluene–hexane–isoamyl alcohol (78:20:2

v/v) (Alternatively, solid-phase extraction techniques have also been reported [15,46].) After mixing and centrifugation, the organic layer was collected and evaporated to dryness under a stream of warm nitrogen. The samples were reconstituted in ethyl acetate (50 µL) and BSTFA + 1% TMCS (50 µL), derivatized by heating for 20 min at 100°C, and transferred to autosampler vials for analysis.

4.2.2. GC/MS Conditions

Chromatographic separation of the analytes was achieved using a 15 m × 0.32 mm i.d. nonpolar fused silica capillary column with 0.25 µm film thickness. The initial temperature of 160°C was held for 1 min. The temperature was increased to 280°C at a rate of 20°C/min. The final temperature was held for 3 min. The injection port and the transfer line were maintained at 265°C and 280°C, respectively. Methane was used as the CI reagent gas for both PICI and NICI analyses. The ionizer pressure was held at 0.5 torr and the analyzer pressure was adjusted to 3.4×10^{-5} torr. The ionizer temperature was maintained at 100°C.

4.2.3. Method Performance

The authors reported a signal-to-noise ratio of 547 at m/z 302 for derivatized and unextracted standards of lorazepam using NICI detection. No observable signal was obtained by PICI or EI for these standards. When urine extracts are analyzed, a limit of quantitation of 10 ng/mL was reported for lorazepam with a %CV of 6.1. Interassay precision on three separate analysis days showed % CVs of 17 and 14 for two different sets of quality control samples.

4.3. Additional Techniques

A method utilizing GC/MS/MS for the analysis of lorazepam in plasma and urine has been reported (43). This method used solid-phase extraction and TMS derivatization of the lorazepam. EI MS/MS analysis was performed using an ion trap MS/MS. Precursor ions for lorazepam–TMS (m/z 429.2) and the internal standard (i.s.), oxazepam-d_5-TMS (m/z 434.2) were fragmented using collision-induced dissociation. Data from three fragment ions were acquired and used for the quantitation and identification of the analytes. The authors reported extraction efficiencies >85% for lorazepam and a limit of quantitation of 0.1 ng/mL in both urine and plasma. Assay precision was not reported.

Few LC/MS methods for the analysis of lorazepam have been reported. Kanazawa et al. (47) described a method using chiral chromatography for the separation of lorazepam enantiomers (47). Although separation of the two enantiomers was achieved, no details were given about the sensitivity of this method.

5. TRIAZOLAM

5.1. Background

Triazolam is a 1,4-triazolo analog of the benzodiazepines and is similar in structure to alprazolam (Fig. 1). In the United States, triazolam is available as 0.125- or 0.25-mg tablets. It is prescribed in doses from 0.125 to a maximum of 0.5 mg/d and is used as a sedative–hypnotic *(4)*. Following oral administration, triazolam is rapidly absorbed and peak plasma concentrations are reached within 2–4 h after administration *(42)*. After a single 0.25-mg dose of triazolam was administered to six subjects, a mean peak plasma concentration of 3.0 ng/mL was attained *(42)*. Triazolam is extensively metabolized, and its principal metabolites are α-hydroxytriazolam and 4-hydroxytriazolam *(48)*. Pharmacokinetic studies indicate that the α-hydroxytriazolam is nearly equipotent to triazolam *(49,50)*. Only about 2% of a dose is eliminated in the urine as triazolam, 70% as α-hydroxytriazolam glucuronide, and 10% as 4-hydroxytriazolam glucuronide *(51)*.

In general, commercial immunoassays have poor cross-reactivity to triazolam and its principal metabolite α-hydroxytriazolam. This, combined with the extremely low therapeutic doses of triazolam and its short plasma half-life (1.5–5.5 h), limit the utility of commercial immunoassays for the detection of triazolam in biological specimens *(4)*. However, it has been demonstrated that conjugated metabolites of triazolam may be detected by on-site testing devices such as Triage™ (Biosite Diagnostics, San Diego, CA) *(2)*. Of the laboratory-based immunoassays, Emit® (Dade Behring, San Jose, CA) was shown to be effective in detecting triazolam use when the urinary concentrations exceeded 100 ng/mL *(2)*. Also, Frazier et al. *(51)* reported that a laboratory-based fluorescence polarization immunoassay was 47% more reactive to α-hydroxytriazolam than to the antibody target drug of nordiazepam *(51)*. Numerous GC methods have been reported for the analysis of triazolam and its metabolites *(2,12)*. As with the analysis of the other benzodiazepine drugs discussed in this chapter, the most effective non-MS methods used ECD *(12)*. For the analysis of triazolam from blood by GC with ECD, the following general method was followed. The blood was extracted under basic conditions with an organic solvent. The reconstituted extraction residues were injected onto either a 15-m methylsilicone or cyanopropylphenyl-fused silica capillary column. A GC temperature program was used *(12)*. The analysis of the hydroxylated metabolites of triazolam by GC required derivatization.

A significant limitation to the analysis of triazolam and α-hydroxytriazolam by GC is the nonvolatile nature of these analytes. Often extended GC temperature programs or very high oven temperatures are needed to elute triazolam and α-hydroxytriazolam from the column.

Triazolam and α-hydroxytriazolam can be analyzed by HPLC *(19–21)*. McIntyre et al. *(20)* used a C18 HPLC column and gradient elution conditions to analyze triazolam in serum, blood, and liver homogenates *(20)*. The recovery of triazolam from blood was 54% and the method was sensitive to 50 ng/mL. Lambert et al. *(21)* used HPLC to analyze triazolam in blood, urine, stomach contents, and various tissue preparations. This method would not be suitable for the analysis of triazolam after single or low therapeutic doses, as sensitivities were in the microgram per milliliter range *(21)*. As with the analysis of alprazolam and its hydroxylated metabolites, HPLC with MS or MS/MS detection are the methods of choice for the analysis of triazolam and α-hydroxytriazolam. These techniques provide improved sensitivity and specificity compared to conventional HPLC methods using UV detection or to EI GC/MS methods.

Several authors have reported methods for the analysis of triazolam and α-hydroxytriazolam using of GC with MS detection *(14,16–18,48,51)*. A typical urine method using EI GC/MS is outlined as follows *(51)*.

1. Add internal standard to 2.0 mL of donor urine, calibrators, and quality control samples.
2. Hydrolyze samples using β-glucronidase at 35°C for 4 h.
3. Make samples basic using a suitable buffer.
4. Extract with methylene chloride.
5. Evaporate organic solvent and derivatize with BSTFA + 1% TMS at 60°C for 30 min.
6. Inject residues onto a 15-m fused silica capillary column at 280°C.

Although the trimethylsilyl derivative is frequently used for the GC analysis of α-hydroxytriazolam, MTBSTFA may be used to form the tertbutyldimethylsilyl derivative. The advantages of this reagent are that it produces higher molecular weight derivatives and that higher *m/z* fragments are formed for EI (or CI) detection. However, extended retention times should be expected. Using a 15-m, 5% phenylpolysiloxane fused silica capillary column and a GC temperature program from 210°C, programmed at a rate of 20°C/min, to a final temperature of 300°C the following relative retention times (RRTs) were observed *(48)*:

Drug	RRT
Oxazepam	1.00
Temazepam	1.08
Lorazepam	1.16
α-Hydroxyalprazolam	1.61
α-Hydroxytriazolam	1.77

5.2. Method 1

CI GC/MS is more selective and sensitive than conventional EI GC/MS for the analysis of triazolam and α-hydroxytriazolam *(17,18)*. Outlined in the following subsections is an unpublished PICI GC/MS method for the analysis of triazolam and α-hydroxytriazolam. The method has been used for the analysis of these (as well as several other benzodiazipines) drugs in plasma and whole blood. This method was modified and published as the NICI method for the analysis of alprazolam presented in an earlier section *(9)*.

5.2.1. Extraction

Calibration curves for triazolam and α-hydroxytriazolam were fortified into plasma or whole blood at concentrations of 0, 2.5, 5.0, 10.0, 25.0, 50.0, 100, 200, 400, and 500 ng/mL. Twenty-five nanograms of triazolam-d_4 and α-hydroxytriazolam-d_4 were added as internal standards. The tubes were mixed, allowed to equilibrate, made basic, and samples were extracted with 7 mL of toluene–methylene chloride (7:3) as previously described. The organic phase was transferred, evaporated, and the residues were reconstituted in 25 μL of ethyl acetate followed by 25 μL of BSTFA + 1% TMCS. The tubes were heated at 80°C for at least 30 min to derivatize the α-hydroxytriazolam.

5.2.2. GC/MS Conditions

Methane and ammonia (approx 4:1) were used as the PICI regent gases. The MS was programmed to acquire SIM data for the following *m/z*: triazolam, 343; triazolam-d_4, 347; α-hydroxytriazolam, 431; and α-hydroxytriazolam-d_4, 435. A 15-m capillary column with a 0.25 mm i.d., 0.25 μm film thickness was used with helium as the carrier gas. The initial GC temperature of 190°C was held for 1 min, then programmed to 320°C at the rate of 20°/min.

5.2.3. Method Performance

The extraction efficiencies for this method were not determined. However, they can be estimated from those reported previously as α-hydroxytriazolam-d_4 was used as the internal standard in that method *(9)*. Further, several authors have reported combined GC/MS methods for triazolam, alprazolam, and their metabolites, indicating that similar recoveries can be expected for the two drugs *(16–18)*. The method was linear for both triazolam and α-hydroxytriazolam from 2.5 to 500 ng/mL. The major limitation of this method was that sensitivities of 1 ng/mL could not be achieved for triazolam or α-hydroxytriazolam.

5.3. Method 2

NICI has been shown to be more than 1000 times more sensitive than either EI or PICI for the analysis of α-hydroxytriazolam *(17)*. In addition, when extracting only 0.2 mL of blood, sensitivities of 0.5 ng/mL were achieved for α-hydroxytriazolam using NICI GC/MS *(18)*. The NICI method of Fitzgerald et al. *(17)* is described in the following subsections *(17)*.

5.3.1. Extraction

Urine calibration curves contained α-hydroxytriazolam (and other benzodiazepines) at concentrations ranging from 50 to 2000 ng/mL. Two hundred and fifty nanograms of α-hydroxytriazolam-d_4 internal standard was added to each tube. The samples were buffered to pH 5 and hydrolyzed using β-glucuronidase. Following hydrolysis, the samples were made basic by adding saturated sodium borate buffer, pH 9, and extracted with 2 mL of toluene–heptane–isoamyl alcohol (78:20:2). The organic phase was transferred and evaporated under a stream of nitrogen. The residues were reconstituted in 50 µL of ethyl acetate followed by 50 µL of BSTFA + 1% TMS and heated at 100°C for at 20 min to derivatize the α-hydroxytriazolam. The tubes were allowed to cool and the liquid was transferred to autosampler vials for analysis.

5.3.2. GC/MS Conditions

Methane was used as the NICI regent gas. The MS was operated in the full scan mode collecting data from *m/z* 250 to 450. A 15 m × 0.32 mm i.d. dimethylpolysiloxane capillary column was used with helium as the carrier gas. The initial GC temperature of 160°C was held for 1 min, then the GC was programmed to 280°C at the rate of 20°/min. The RRT of α-hydroxytriazolam to oxazepam was 1.71.

5.3.3. Method Performance

The extraction efficiencies for α-hydroxytriazolam at 500 ng/mL was approx 73%. The method was linear for both from 50 to 2000 ng/mL. The precision of the method was experimentally determined at several concentrations in the linear range. For α-hydroxytriazolam, the intraassay precision was <3.1% CV at all concentrations tested. The interassay precision was 21% CV at 131 ng/mL and 3.2% CV at 1086 ng/mL.

References

1. Hardman, J. G., Limbird, L. E., Molinoff, P. B., et al., (Eds.) (1996) *Goodman & Gilman's The Pharmocoligical Basis of Therapeutics*. McGraw-Hill, New York.

2. Drummer, O. H. (1999) Chromatographic screening techniques in systematic toxicological analysis. *J. Chromatogr. B Biomed. Sci. Appl.* **733,** 27–45.
3. Huang, W., Moody, D. E., Andrenyak, D. M, and Rollins, D. E. (1993) Immunoassay detection of nordiazepam, triazolam, lorazepam, and alprazolam in blood. *J. Analyt. Toxicol.* **17,** 365–369.
4. Walsh, P. (Ed). (2000) *Physicians' Desk Reference.* Medical Economics, Montvale, NJ.
5. Kissin, W. and Ball, J. (1999) Year-End 1998 Emergency Department Data from the Drug Abuse Warning Network. SAMHSA, Office of Applied Studies.
6. Greenblatt, D. J., von Moltke, L. L., Harmatz, J. S., et al. (1993) Alprazolam pharmacokinetics, metabolism, and plasma levels: clinical implications. *J. Clin. Psychiatry* **54** (Suppl), 4–11; discussion 12–14.
7. Greenblatt, D. J. and Wright, C. E. (1993) Clinical pharmacokinetics of alprazolam. Therapeutic implications. *Clin. Pharmacokinet.* **24,** 453–471.
8. Crouch, D. J., Rollins, D. E., Canfield, D. V., et al. (1999) Quantitation of alprazolam and alpha-hydroxyalprazolam in human plasma using liquid chromatography electrospray ionization MS-MS. *J. Analyt. Toxicol.* **23,** 479–485.
9. Hold, K. M., Crouch, D. J., and Rollins, D. E. (1996) Determination of alprazolam and alpha-hydroxyalprazolam in human plasma by gas chromatography/negative-ion chemical ionization mass spectrometry. *J. Mass Spectrom.* **31,** 1033–1038.
10. Greenblatt, D. J., Harmatz, J. S., and Shader, R. I. (1993) Plasma alprazolam concentrations. Relation to efficacy and side effects in the treatment of panic disorder. *Arch. Gen. Psychiatry* **50,** 715–722.
11. Greenblatt, D. J., Javaid, J. I., Locniskar, A., et al. (1990) Gas chromatographic analysis of alprazolam in plasma: replicability, stability and specificity. *J. Chromatogr.* **534,** 202–207.
12. Gjerde, H., Dahlin, E., and Christophersen, A. S. (1992) Simultaneous determination of common benzodiazepines in blood using capillary gas chromatography. *J. Pharmaceut. Biomed. Anal.* **10,** 317–322.
13. Greenblatt, D. J. (1992) Pharmacology of benzodiazepine hypnotics. *J. Clin. Psychiatry* **53** (Suppl), 7–13.
14. Maurer, H. and Pfleger, K. (1987) Identification and differentiation of benzodiazepines and their metabolites in urine by computerized gas chromatography-mass spectrometry. *J. Chromatogr.* **422,** 85–101.
15. Black, D. A., Clark, G. D., Haver, V. M., et al. (1994) Analysis of urinary benzodiazepines using solid-phase extraction and gas chromatography-mass spectrometry. *J. Analyt. Toxicol.* **18,** 185–188.
16. Joern, W. A. (1992) Confirmation of low concentrations of urinary benzodiazepines, including alprazolam and triazolam, by GC/MS: an extractive alkylation procedure. *J. Analyt. Toxicol.* **16,** 363–367.
17. Fitzgerald, R. L., Rexin, D. A., and Herold, D. A. (1993) Benzodiazepine analysis by negative chemical ionization gas chromatography/mass spectrometry. *J. Analyt. Toxicol.* **17,** 342–347.
18. Cairns, E. R., Dent, B. R., Ouwerkerk, J. C., and Porter, L. J. (1994) Quantitative analysis of alprazolam and triazolam in hemolysed whole blood and liver digest by GC/MS/NICI with deuterated internal standards. *J. Analyt. Toxicol.* **18,** 1–6.

19. Jin, L. and Lau, C. E. (1994) Determination of alprazolam and its major metabolites in serum microsamples by high-performance liquid chromatography and its application to pharmacokinetics in rats. *J. Chromatogr. B Biomed. Appl.* **654,** 77–83.
20. McIntyre, I. M., Norman, T. R., Burrows, G. D., and Armstrong, S. M. (1993) Alterations to plasma melatonin and cortisol after evening alprazolam administration in humans. *Chronobiol. Int.* **10,** 205–213.
21. Lambert, W. E., Meyer, E. Y., Xue-Ping, and De Leenheer, A. P. (1995) Screening, identification, and quantitation of benzodiazepines in postmortem samples by HPLC with photodiode array detection. *J. Analyt. Toxicol.* **19,** 35–40.
22. Kleinschnitz, M., Herderich, M., and Schreier, P. (1996) Determination of 1,4-benzodiazepines by high-performance liquid chromatography-electrospray tandem mass spectrometry. *J. Chromatogr. B Biomed. Appl.* **676,** 61–67.
23. Greenblatt, D. J. and Shader, R. I. (1984) Short half-life benzodiazepines. *Ration. Drug Ther.* **18,** 1–5.
24. Jones, C. E., Wians, F. H. Jr., Martinez, L. A., and Merritt, G. J. (1989) Benzodiazepines screening used to detect benzophenone derivatives. *Clin. Chem.* **35,** 1394–1398.
25. Augsburger, M., Rivier, L., and Mangin, P. (1998) Comparison of different immunoassays and GC-MS screening of benzodiazepines in urine. *J. Pharmaceut. Biomed. Anal.* **18,** 681–687.
26. Bourget, P., Bouton, V., Lesne-Hulin, A., et al. (1996) Comparison of high-performance liquid chromatography and polyclonal fluorescence polarization immunoassay for the monitoring of midazolam in the plasma of intensive care unit patients. *Ther. Drug Monit.* **18,** 610–619.
27. Fitzgerald, R. L., Rexin, D. A., and Herold, D. A. (1994) Detecting benzodiazepines: immunoassays compared with negative chemical ionization gas chromatography/mass spectrometry. *Clin. Chem.* **40,** 373–380.
28. Way, B. A., Walton, K. G., Koenig, J. W., et al. (1998) Comparison between the CEDIA and EMIT II immunoassays for the determination of benzodiazepines. *Clin. Chim. Acta.* **271,** 1–9.
29. Nishikawa, T., Ohtani, H., Herold, D. A., and Fitzgerald, R. L. (1997) Comparison of assay methods for benzodiazepines in urine. A receptor assay, two immunoassays, and gas chromatography-mass spectrometry. *Am. J. Clin. Pathol.* **107,** 345–352.
30. Schafroth, M., Thormann, W., and Allemann, D. (1994) Micellar electrokinetic capillary chromatography of benzodiazepines in human urine. *Electrophoresis* **15,** 72–78.
31. Beyer, R. and Seyde, W. C. (1992) Propofol versus midazolam. Long-term sedation in the intensive care unit. *Anaesthesist* **41,** 335–341.
32. Martens, J. and Banditt, P. (1997) Simultaneous determination of midazolam and its metabolites 1-hydroxymidazolam and 4-hydroxymidazolam in human serum using gas chromatography-mass spectrometry. *J. Chromatogr. B Biomed. Sci. Appl.* **692,** 95–100.
33. de Vries, J. X., Rudi, J., Walter-Sack, I., and Conradi, R. (1990) The determination of total and unbound midazolam in human plasma. A comparison of high performance liquid chromatography, gas chromatography and gas chromatography/mass spectrometry. *Biomed. Chromatogr.* **4,** 28–33.

34. Lee, T. C. and Charles, B. (1996) The determination of total and unbound midazolam in human plasma. A comparison of high performance liquid chromatography, gas chromatography and gas chromatography/mass spectrometry. *Biomed. Chromatogr.* **10,** 65–68.
35. Ha, H. R., Rentsch, K. M., Kneer, J., and Vonderschmitt, D. J. (1993) Determination of midazolam and its alpha-hydroxy metabolite in human plasma and urine by high-performance liquid chromatography. *Ther. Drug Monit.* **15,** 338–343.
36. Puglisi, C. V., Pao, J., Ferrara, F. J., and de Silva, J. A. (1985) Determination of midazolam and its alpha-hydroxy metabolite in human plasma and urine high-performance liquid chromatography. *J. Chromatogr.* **344,** 199–209.
37. Portier, E. J., de Blok, K., Butter, J. J., and van Boxtel, C. J. (1999) Simultaneous determination of fentanyl and midazolam using high-performance liquid chromatography with ultraviolet detection. *J. Chromatogr. B Biomed. Sci. Appl.* **723,** 313–318.
38. Kanazawa, H., Nagata, Y., Matsushima, Y., et al. (1993) Liquid chromatography-mass spectrometry for the determination of medetomidine and other anaesthetics in plasma. *J. Chromatogr.* **631,** 215–220.
39. Marquet, P., Baudin, O., Gaulier, J. M., et al. (1999) Sensitive and specific determination of midazolam and 1-hydroxymidazolam in human serum by liquid chromatography-electrospray mass spectrometry. *J. Chromatogr. B Biomed. Sci. Appl.* **734,** 137–144.
40. Lausecker, B., Hopfgartner, G., and Hesse, M. (1998) Capillary electrophoresis-mass spectrometry coupling versus micro-high-performance liquid chromatography-mass spectrometry coupling: a case study. *J. Chromatogr. B Biomed. Sci. Appl.* **718,** 1–13.
41. Greenblatt, D. J., Schillings, R. T., Kyriakopoulos, A. A., et al. (1976) Clinical pharmacokinetics of lorazepam. I. Absorption and disposition of oral 14C-lorazepam. *Clin. Pharmacol. Ther.* **20,** 329–341.
42. Baselt, R. C. and Cravey, R. H. (1995) *Disposition of Toxic Drugs and Chemicals in Man*, 4th edit., Chemical Toxicology Institute, Foster City, CA.
43. Pichini, S., Pacifici, R., Altieri, I., et al. (1999). Determination of lorazepam in plasma and urine as trimethylsilyl derivative using gas chromatography-tandem mass spectrometry. *J. Chromatogr. B Biomed. Sci. Appl.* **732,** 509–514.
44. Higuchi, S., Urabe, H., and Shiobara, Y. (1979) Simplified determination of lorazepam and oxazepam in biological fluids by gas chromatography-mass spectrometry. *J. Chromatogr.* **164,** 55–61.
45. Meatherall, R. (1994). GC-MS confirmation of urinary benzodiazepine metabolites. *J. Analyt. Toxicol.* **18,** 369–381.
46. Koves, E. M. and Yen, B. (1989) The use of gas chromatography/negative ion chemical ionization mass spectrometry for the determination of lorazepam in whole blood. *J. Analyt. Toxicol.* **13,** 69–72.
47. Kanazawa, H., Konishi, Y., Matsushima, Y., and Takahashi, T. (1998) Determination of with a desalting system. *J. Chromatogr. A* **797,** 227–236.
48. Dickson, P. H., Markus, W., McKernan, J., and Nipper, H. C. (1992). Urinalysis of alpha-hydroxyalprazolam, alpha-hydroxytriazolam, and other benzodiazepine compounds by GC/EIMS. *J. Analyt. Toxicol.* **16,** 67–71.

49. Pakes, G. E., Brogden, R. N., Heel, R. C., et al. (1981). Triazolam: a review of its pharmacological properties and therapeutic efficacy in patients with insomnia. *Drugs* **22,** 81–110.
50. Fraser, A. D. (1987) Urinary screening for alprazolam, triazolam, and their metabolites with the EMIT d.a.u. benzodiazepine metabolite assay. *J. Analyt. Toxicol.* **11,** 263–266.
51. Fraser, A. D., Bryan, W., and Isner, A. F. (1992) Urinary screening for alpha-OH triazolam by FPIA and EIA with confirmation by GC/MS. *J. Analyt. Toxicol.* **16,** 347–350.

Chapter 5

Identification of Benzodiazepines in Human Hair
A Review

Vincent Cirimele and Pascal Kintz

1. INTRODUCTION

Benzodiazepines are the most commonly prescribed drugs in the world, in part because of their efficacy, safety, and low cost. They are prescribed for their anxiolytic, sedative, hypnotic, anticonvulsant, and muscle relaxant properties. They are also the most abused pharmaceuticals, so they occur more frequently than any type of drug in overdose cases. Fortunately, however, they are relatively safe drugs, even at overdose concentrations, apparently because of rapid body adaptation to high blood levels. Nevertheless, they may have a synergistic effect when taken with alcohol and other drugs such as morphinomimetics, antidepressants, sedatives, or neuroleptics.

Generally, drug testing is based on blood or urine measurement, but blood concentration may only reflect dosage at the time of sampling. To assess exposure over longer periods, it would be an advantage to sample a readily accessible tissue, which provides a more permanent marker of drug intake. To obtain data on individual past history of chronic dosage, drug analysis of hair was suggested to be useful *(1)*. More recently, it was demonstrated that a single 2-mg Rohypnol® administration can be revealed by 7-amino-flunitrazepam detection in hair when tested 24 h later *(2)*.

From: *Forensic Science: Benzodiazepines and GHB: Detection and Pharmacology*
Edited by: S. J. Salamone © Humana Press Inc., Totowa, NJ

Technically, testing of hair for drugs is no more difficult or challenging than testing in many other matrices (e.g., liver, bone, etc.). In fact, the applications of analytical methods and instrumental approaches are in most cases quite similar, regardless of the initial matrix.

Since the early 1980s, the development of highly sensitive and sensitive analytical methods such as radioimmunoassay (RIA) or gas chromatography/mass spectrometry (GC/MS) has allowed the determination of organic, exogenous compounds trapped in hair.

During 1980–90, particular attention had been given to the use of hair for the detection of drugs of abuse such as cocaine, heroin, amphetamines, and cannabis. However, the detection in human hair of benzodiazepines, the most abused pharmaceutical drugs in the world, appeared later.

The present chapter aims to review the articles devoted to the detection of these compounds in hair.

2. BIOLOGY OF HAIR

Hair is a product of differentiated organs in the skin of mammals. It differs in individuals only in color, quantity, and texture. Hair seems to be a vestigial structure in humans, as it is too sparse to provide protection against cold or trauma.

Hair composition is primarily protein (65–95%, keratin essentially), and also water (15–35%) and lipids (1–9%). The mineral content of hair ranges from 0.25 to 0.95%. The total number of hair follicles in an adult human is estimated to be about 5 million, with 1 million found on the head *(3)*. Hair follicles are embedded in the epidermal epithelium of the skin, approx 3–4 mm below the skin's surface.

Each hair shaft consists of an outer cuticle that surrounds a cortex. The cortex may contain a central medulla. The hair follicle is closely associated with two glands: the sebaceous gland, which secretes sebum (a fatty substance), and the apocrine gland, which secretes an oily substance. The ducts of these two glands empty into the follicle.

2.1. Hair Growth

Hair shafts originate in cells located in a germination center, called the matrix, located at the base of the follicle. Hair does not grow continually, but in cycles, alternating between periods of growth and quiescence. A follicle that is actively producing hair is said to be in the *anagen* phase. Scalp hair has the greatest variability in growth rate, but also the highest one. Growth rates range from 0.2 to 1.12 mm/d. The growth/rest cycle for scalp hair is short (30 mo/

3–2.5 mo on average), especially in the vertex region, where 85% of the follicles are in the anagen phase. Beard hairs have the lowest growth rate (approx 0.27 mm/d) and a long growth/rest cycle duration of 14–22 mo/9–12 mo. Axillary and pubic hairs are quite similar in terms of growth rate (approx 0.3 mm/d) and growth/rest cycle durations (11–18 mo/12–17 mo) *(4)*. After this period, the follicle enters a relatively short transition period of about 2 wk, known as the *catagen* phase, during which cell division stops and the follicle begins to degenerate. Following the transition phase, the hair follicle enters a resting or quiescent period, known as the *telogen* phase (10 wk), in which the hair shaft stops growing completely and the hair begins to shut down.

Factors such as race, disease states, nutritional deficiencies, and age are known to influence both the rate of growth and the length of the quiescent period. On the scalp of an adult, approx 85% of the hair is in the growing phase and the remaining 15% is in a resting stage.

When hair shafts grow, they move up the follicle into the keratinogeneous zone, where they synthesize melanin and keratin. Melanin is synthesized from tyrosine in the melanocytes, while keratin is formed from a special protein of high sulfur content.

2.2. Types of Hair

Pubic hair, arm hair, and axillary hair have been suggested as an alternative source for drug detection when scalp hair is not available. Various studies have found differences in concentrations between pubic or axillary hair and scalp hair. The significant differences of the drug concentrations were explained on the basis of a better blood circulation, a greater number of apocrine glands, a totally different telogen/anagen ratio, and a different growth rate of the hair.

2.3. Mechanisms of Drug Incorporation into Hair

It is generally proposed that drugs can enter into hair by two processes: adsorption from the external environment and incorporation into the growing hair shaft from blood supplying the hair follicle. Drugs can enter the hair from exposure to chemicals in aerosols, smoke, or secretions from sweat and sebaceous glands. Sweat is known to contain drugs present in blood. Because hair is very porous and can increase in weight up to 18% by absorbing liquids, drugs may be transferred easily to hair via sweat. Finally, chemicals present in air (smoke, vapors, etc.) can be deposited onto hair.

The model generally proposed for the incorporation of drugs into hair is one in which drugs are transferred passively from the blood into the growing cells of the hair follicle and become trapped during keratogenesis (the formation of keratin). However, the biology of hair is too complex to support this model.

Drugs appear to be incorporated into the hair during at least three stages: from the blood during hair formation, from sweat and sebum, and from the external environment. This model is more capable than a passive model of exlaining several experimental findings such as: (1) Drug and metabolite ratios in blood are quite different than those found in hair and (2) drug and metabolite concentrations in hair differ markedly in individuals receiving the same dose. Evidence for the transfer of the drug via sweat and sebum can be supported, as drugs and metabolites are present in sweat and sebum at high concentrations and persist in these secretions longer than they do in blood. The parent drug can be found in sweat long after it has disappeared from the blood.

The exact mechanism by which chemicals are bound to hair is not known. It has been suggested that passive diffusion may be augmented by drug binding to intracellular components of the hair cells such as the hair pigment melanin. This is an especially attractive mechanism for drugs such as amphetamine and methamphetamine, which are chemically similar to tyrosine and dihydroxyphenylalanine (DOPA), the precursors of melanin. However, this is probably not an important mechanism because drugs are trapped into the hair of albino animals, which lack melanin. Another augmenting mecanism proposed is the binding of drugs with sulfhydryl-containing amino acids present in hair. There is an abundance of amino acids such as cystine in hair that form crosslinking S–S bonds to stabilize the protein fiber network *(3)*. Drugs diffusing into hair cells could be bound in this way.

2.4. Effects of Cosmetic Treatments

An important issue of concern for drug analysis in hair is the change in the drug concentration induced by cosmetic treatment of hair. Hair is continuously subjected to natural factors, such as sunlight, weather, water, pollution, and so forth, that affect and damage the cuticle but hair cosmetic treatments enhance that damage. Particular attention has been focused on the effects of repeated shampooing, perming, relaxing, and dyeing of hair. After cosmetic treatments (bleaching), benzodiazepine concentrations decline dramatically, decreasing by 39.7%, 67.7%, and 61.8% of the original concentration of diazepam, nordazepam, and 7-amino-flunitrazepam, respectively *(5)*. The products used for cosmetic treatments, such as bleaching, permanent waving, dyeing, or relaxing, are strong bases. They will cause hair damage and affect drug content (by loss) or affect directly drug stability.

3. Specimen Collection

Collection procedures for hair analysis for drugs have not been standardized. In most published studies, the samples are obtained from random locations on the scalp. Hair is best collected from the area at the back of the head, called the *vertex posterior*. Compared with other areas of the head, this area has less variability in hair growth rate, the number of hairs in the growing phase is more constant, and the hair is less subject to age- and sex-related influences.

The sample size varies considerably among laboratories and depends on the drug to be analyzed and the test methodology. Sample sizes reported in the literature range from 3 to 80 mg (Table 1).

Multisectional analysis involves taking a length of hair and cutting it into sections to measure drug use during shorter periods of time (segments of about 1, 2, or 3 cm, which correspond to about 1, 2, or 3 months' growth). The hair must be cut as close as possible to the scalp. Particular care is also required to ensure that the individual hairs in the cutoff tuft retain the position they originally had beside one another. It has been claimed that this technique can be applied to provide a retrospective calendar of an individual's drug use. For example, a sectional analysis was performed on a hair strand of 16 cm long to demonstrate an increased self-medication with lorazepam *(18)*.

4. Decontamination Procedures

Most laboratories use a wash step (Table 1); however, there is no consensus or uniformity in the washing procedures. Generally, a single washing step is realized; sometimes a second identical wash is performed. Among the agents used in washing are aqueous solutions or organic solvents.

5. Extraction

In all the cases, the hair strand is pulverized in a ball mill, cut into small segments (approx 1 mm in length), or used in its entirety. To determine the amount of a drug in hair, it is necessary to solubilize the drugs. Various drug solubilization methods have been proposed, including chemical (acid or base) extraction, organic solvent extraction, or enzymatic digestion, but this step must be such that the analytes are not altered or lost. The alkaline or acid hydrolyses of hair are not suitable for the extraction of chemically unstable compounds such as benzodiazepines because they lead to the formation of benzophenones. Large series of results were obtained using incubation in buffer such as Soerensen buffer or an acetate buffer with β-glucuronidase-arylsulfatase (Table 2).

Table 1
Preparation of the Hair Specimens

Drug	Weight	Wash procedure	Reference
Flunitrazepam, 7-amino-flunitrazepam	50 mg	Water	2
Diazepam, nordiazepam, 7-amino-flunitrazepam	30 mg	Warm water (5 min) and acetone (1 min)	5
Diazepam, nordiazepam, flunitrazepam, nitrazepam	50 mg	Ethanol, 15 min at 37°C	6
Diazepam	3 mg	Ethanol and phosphate buffer at 37°C	7
Diazepam, nordiazepam	50 mg	Ethanol, 15 min at 37°C	8
Diazepam, nordiazepam, flunitrazepam, nitrazepam	50 mg	Ethanol, 15 min at 37°C	9
Diazepam, nordiazepam, flunitrazepam, nitrazepam	50 mg	Ethanol, 15 min at 37°C	10
Diazepam, oxazepam	50 mg	Methylene chloride, 15 min at 37°C	11
Diazepam, oxazepam	50 mg	Methylene chloride, 15 min at 37°C	12
Nordiazepam[a]	25–50 mg	Water, acetone and n-hexane	13
Clobazam	50 mg	Ethanol	14
Nordiazepam, oxazepam	50 mg	Methylene chloride	15
Diazepam, nitrazepam, oxazepam	5–25 mg	Water and methanol	16
Benzodiazepines	10 mg	Methylene chloride	17
Lorazepam	50 mg	Methylene chloride	18
Flunitrazepam, 7-amino-flunitrazepam	50 mg	Methylene chloride	19
Alprazolam	80 mg	Methylene chloride and phosphate buffer	20
Flunitrazepam, 7-amino-flunitrazepam	50 mg	Methylene chloride	21
Nordiazepam, oxazepam, bromazepam, diazepam, lorazepam, flunitrazepam, alprazolam, triazolam	50 mg	Methylene chloride	22
Nordiazepam, oxazepam, lormetazepam, lorazepam, diazepam, 7-amino-flunitrazepam	30–50 mg	Warm water and acetone	23
Flunitrazepam, 7-amino-flunitrazepam	50 mg	Water	24

[a]Added to negative hair specimens.

Table 2
Solubilization of Benzodiazepines from Hair

Drug	Hydrolysis	Reference
Flunitrazepam, 7-amino-flunitrazepam	Ultrasonic bath in methanol for 1 h and 0.1 M HCl, overnight at 55°C	2
Diazepam, nordiazepam, 7-amino-flunitrazepam	8 M urea–0.2 M thioglycolate, pH 3.0, 2 h at 60°C	5
Diazepam, nordiazepam, flunitrazepam, nitrazepam	1 M NaOH, 10 min at 100°C	6
Diazepam	Not published	7
Diazepam, nordiazepam	1 M NaOH, 10 min at 100°C	8
Diazepam, nordiazepam, flunitrazepam, nitrazepam	1 M NaOH, 10 min at 100°C	9
Diazepam, nordiazepam, flunitrazepam, nitrazepam	1 M NaOH, 10 min at 100°C	10
Diazepam, oxazepam	1 M NaOH, 10 min at 100°C	11
Diazepam, oxazepam	1 M HCl, 12 h at 50°C	12
Nordiazepam	Ultrasonic bath in acetone for 2 h, then 12 h at 40°C	13
Clobazam	0.1 M HCl, 12 h at 56°C	14
Nordiazepam, oxazepam	Soerensen buffer, 20 h at 40°C	15
Diazepam, nitrazepam, oxazepam	Methanol, 18 h at 55°C	16
Benzodiazepines	Methanol/trifluoroacetic acid (9:1, v/v), overnight at 37°C	17
Lorazepam	Soerensen buffer, 2 h at 40°C	18
Flunitrazepam, 7-amino-flunitrazepam	Soerensen buffer, 2 h at 40°C	19
Alprazolam	0.1M HCl, 12 h at 56°C	20
Flunitrazepam, 7-amino-flunitrazepam	Soerensen buffer, 2 h at 40°C	21
Nordiazepam, oxazepam, bromazepam, diazepam, lorazepam, flunitrazepam, alprazolam, triazolam	Soerensen buffer, 2 h at 40°C	22
Nordiazepam, oxazepam, lormetazepam, lorazepam, diazepam, 7-amino-flunitrazepam	β-glucuronidase-arylsulfatase, 2 h at 40°C	23
Flunitrazepam, 7-amino-flunitrazepam	Ultrasonic bath in methanol for 1 h and 0.1M HCl, overnight at 55°C	24

Different extraction procedures are used to purify the benzodiazepine compounds solubilized from hair (Table 3), but liquid–liquid processes are preferred in contrast with solid-phase extraction on columns. The development and use of deuterated internal standards (possible only with mass selective detectors) permit an easier and more accurate quantification of the target drugs (Table 3).

6. DETECTION

One article reports the detection of target drugs by radioimmunoassay *(7)*. Diazepam was readily detected, but alprazolam and lorazepam were not found in subjects receiving therapeutic dosages.

Chromatographic procedures seems to be a more powerful tool for the identification and quantification of drugs in hair, owing to their separation ability and their detection sensibility. In 1995, Couper et al. *(16)* established a procedure for the detection of psychotic drugs in hair by high-performance liquid chromatography (HPLC), but diazepam, nitrazepam, and oxazepam were not detected in hair samples from subjects under treatment. Classical HPLC was certainly inadequate for the detection of benzodiazepines in human hair owing to a lack of sensitivity.

In most cases, GC/MS in either electron ionization (EI) or negative chemical ionization (NCI) mode was used (Table 4). The GC/MS examination is carried out in each case without derivatization or after derivatization either by sylilation or acylation. However, to detect diazepam, nitrazepam, and oxazepam *(16)*, or alprazolam *(20)*, liquid chromatography with UV detection (HPLC/UV), gas chromatography with electron capture detection (GC/ECD), or liquid chromatography with diode array detection (HPLC/DAD), respectively, were employed. Enzyme-linked immunosorbent assay (ELISA) test was used in only one case *(17)*. The limitations of this technique were the absence of specific identification of the drug and the approximative quantification (in equivalent diazepam). The analytical detection limits of each technique are summarized in Table 5. For GC/MS, they ranged from 0.2 to 250 pg/mg. GC/MS/NCI represents the state-of-the-art to test benzodiazepines in human hair, owing to the high electrophilic character of the analytes. Benzodiazepines possess halogen groups (electronegative functional groups) located on aromatic rings with high negative density that will give more stability to the anions formed in the ion source.

As demonstrated by the quantitative levels found (Table 6), benzodiazepine concentrations are generally low. Some of them were detected in the nanogram per milligram range (nordiazepam, diazepam, oxazepam) where some

Table 3
Purification Procedures

Drug	IS	Extraction	Reference
Flunitrazepam, 7-amino-flunitrazepam	Deuterated analogs	Solid-phase extraction	2
Diazepam, nordiazepam, 7-amino-flunitrazepam	Deuterated analogs	Solid-phase extraction	5
Diazepam, nordiazepam, flunitrazepam, nitrazepam	SKF 525A	Chloroform–2-propanol–n-heptane (50:17:33, v/v/v)	6
Diazepam	None	Not published	7
Diazepam, nordiazepam	SKF 525A	Chloroform–2-propanol–n-heptane (50:17:33, v/v/v)	8
Diazepam, nordiazepam, flunitrazepam, nitrazepam	SKF 525A	Chloroform–2-propanol–n-heptane (50:17:33, v/v/v)	9
Diazepam, nordiazepam, flunitrazepam, nitrazepam	SKF 525A	Chloroform–2-propanol–n-heptane (50:17:33, v/v/v)	10
Diazepam, oxazepam	Not published	Chloroform–2-propanol–n-heptane (50:17:33, v/v/v)	11
Diazepam, oxazepam	Not published	Chloroform–2-propanol–n-heptane (50:17:33, v/v/v)	12
Nordiazepam	None	None	13
Clobazam	Diazepam	Diethylether–chloroform (80:20, v/v)	14
Nordiazepam, oxazepam	Deuterated analogs	Diethylether–chloroform (80:20, v/v)	15
Diazepam, nitrazepam, oxazepam	Clobazam	Chlorobutane, pH 9.5, and orthophosphoric acid	16
Benzodiazepines	None	None	17
Lorazepam	Lorazepam-d_4	Diethylether–chloroform (80:20, v/v)	18
Flunitrazepam, 7-amino-flunitrazepam	Diazepam-d_5	Diethylether–chloroform (80:20, v/v)	19
Alprazolam	Not published	Solid-phase extraction	20
Flunitrazepam, 7-amino-flunitrazepam	Diazepam-d_5	Diethylether–chloroform (80:20, v/v)	21
Nordiazepam, oxazepam, bromazepam, diazepam, lorazepam, flunitrazepam, alprazolam, triazolam	Prazepam-d_5	Diethylether–chloroform (80:20, v/v)	22
Nordiazepam, oxazepam, lormetazepam, lorazepam, diazepam, 7-amino-flunitrazepam	Deuterated analogs	Solid-phase extraction	23
Flunitrazepam, 7-amino-flunitrazepam	Deuterated analogs	Solid-phase extraction	24

IS, Internal standard.

Table 4
Derivation Step and Detection Techniques

Drug	Derivation	Detection	Reference
Flunitrazepam, 7-amino-flunitrazepam	HFBA	GC/MS–NCI	2
Diazepam, nordiazepam, 7-amino-flunitrazepam	HFBA	GC/MS–EI	5
Diazepam, nordiazepam, flunitrazepam, nitrazepam	None	GC/MS–EI	6
Diazepam	None	RIA	7
Diazepam, nordiazepam	None	GC/MS–EI	8
Diazepam, nordiazepam, flunitrazepam, nitrazepam	None	GC/MS–EI	9
Diazepam, nordiazepam, flunitrazepam, nitrazepam	None	GC/MS–EI	10
Diazepam, oxazepam	None	GC/MS–EI	11
Diazepam, oxazepam	None	GC/MS–EI	12
Nordiazepam	None	RIA and KIMS-immunoassay	13
Clobazam	BSTFA (1% TMCS)	GC/MS–EI	14
Nordiazepam, oxazepam	BSTFA (1% TMCS)	GC/MS–NCI	15
Diazepam, nitrazepam, oxazepam	None	HPLC–UV	16
Benzodiazepines	None	ELISA test	17
Lorazepam	BSTFA (1% TMCS)	GC/MS–NCI	18
Flunitrazepam, 7-amino-flunitrazepam	HFBA	GC/MS–NCI	19
Alprazolam	None	HPLC–DAD and GC/MS–EI	20
Flunitrazepam, 7-amino-flunitrazepam	HFBA	GC/MS–NCI	21
Nordiazepam, oxazepam, bromazepam, diazepam, lorazepam, flunitrazepam, alprazolam, triazolam	BSTFA (1% TMCS)	GC/MS–NCI	22
Nordiazepam, oxazepam, lormetazepam, lorazepam, diazepam, 7-amino-flunitrazepam	None	GC/MS–EI	23
Flunitrazepam, 7-amino-flunitrazepam	HFBA	GC/MS–NCI	24

Table 5
Sensitivity of the Established Procedures

Drug	Detection limit	Reference
Flunitrazepam, 7-amino-flunitrazepam	1.5 and 0.2 pg/mg	2
Diazepam, nordiazepam, 7-amino-flunitrazepam	0.02–0.08 ng/mg	5
Diazepam, nordiazepam, flunitrazepam, nitrazepam	Not published	6
Diazepam	0.15 ng/mg	7
Diazepam, nordiazepam	0.03–0.1 ng/mg	8
Diazepam, nordiazepam, flunitrazepam, nitrazepam	0.03–0.1 ng/mg	9
Diazepam, nordiazepam, flunitrazepam, nitrazepam	0.03–0.1 ng/mg	10
Diazepam, oxazepam	0.1 ng/mg	11
Diazepam, oxazepam	0.1 ng/mg	12
Nordiazepam	KIMS 0.2 ng/mg/RIA 0.1 ng/mg	13
Clobazam	Not published	14
Nordiazepam, oxazepam	10 pg/mg	15
Diazepam, nitrazepam, oxazepam	0.1–0.25 ng/mg	16
Benzodiazepines	Not published	17
Lorazepam	2 pg/mg	18
Flunitrazepam, 7-amino-flunitrazepam	15 pg/mg and 3 pg/mg	19
Alprazolam	Not published	20
Flunitrazepam, 7-amino-flunitrazepam	15 pg/mg and 3 pg/mg	21
Nordiazepam, oxazepam, bromazepam, diazepam, lorazepam, flunitrazepam, alprazolam, triazolam	1–20 pg/mg	22
Nordiazepam, oxazepam, lormetazepam, lorazepam, diazepam, 7-amino-flunitrazepam	Not published	23
Flunitrazepam, 7-amino-flunitrazepam	1.5 and 0.2 pg/mg	24

Table 6
Analytical Results

Drug	Tested	Positive	Range concentration	Mean	Reference
Flunitrazepam	10	Not published	Not published	Not published	2
7-Amino-flunitrazepam	10	Not published	Not published	Not published	
Diazepam	2	2	0.06 and 0.04 ng/mg[a]	—	5
Nordiazepam	2	2	0.99 and 0.32 ng/mg[a]	—	
7-Amino-flunitrazepam	2	2	0.06 and not detected[a]	—	
Diazepam	Not published	1	1.37 ng/mg	—	6
Nordiazepam	Not published	2	1.04 and 1.47 ng/mg	1.26 ng/mg	
Flunitrazepam	Not published	1	0.41 ng/mg	—	
Nitrazepam	Not published	1	0.37 ng/mg	—	
Diazepam	14	12	0.2–1.64 ng/mg	0.53 ng/mg	7
Diazepam	54	1	1.37 ng/mg	—	8
Nordiazepam	54	2	1.04 and 1.47 ng/mg	1.26 ng/mg	
Diazepam	Not published	1	1.37 ng/mg	—	9
Nordiazepam	Not published	3	1.04–2.41 ng/mg	1.64 ng/mg	
Flunitrazepam	Not published	1	0.41 ng/mg	—	
Nitrazepam	Not published	1	0.37 ng/mg	—	
Diazepam	40	1	1.37 ng/mg	—	10
Nordiazepam	40	3	1.04–2.41 ng/mg	1.64 ng/mg	
Flunitrazepam	40	1	0.41 ng/mg	—	
Nitrazepam	40	1	0.37 ng/mg	—	
Diazepam	11	8	3.36–17.55 ng/mg	Not published	11
Oxazepam	11	3	0.78–31.83 ng/mg	Not published	
Diazepam	11	8	3.36–17.55 ng/mg	Not published	12
Oxazepam	11	3	0.78–31.83 ng/mg	Not published	
Nordiazepam	No real hair	—	—	—	13
Clobazam	1	1	6.28 ng/mg	—	14

Compound			Range	Value	Ref
Nordiazepam	30	13	0.25–18.90 ng/mg	4.16 ng/mg	15
Oxazepam	30	5	0.11–0.50 ng/mg	0.28 ng/mg	
Diazepam	3	0	—	—	16
Nitrazepam	3	0	—	—	
Oxazepam	3	0	—	—	
Benzodiazepines	81	—	0.04–0.23 diazepam equivalent	Not published	17
Lorazepam	4	4	31–49 pg/mg	40 pg/mg	18
Flunitrazepam	1	1	89.5 pg/mg	—	19
7-Amino-flunitrazepam	1	1	24 pg/mg	—	
Alprazolam	1	1	0.3 ng/mg	—	20
Flunitrazepam	40	14	31–129 pg/mg	60 pg/mg	21
7-Amino-flunitrazepam	40	26	3–161 pg/mg	46 pg/mg	
Nordiazepam	115	42	0.20–18.87 ng/mg	4.78 ng/mg	
Oxazepam	115	14	0.10–0.50 ng/mg	0.35 ng/mg	
Bromazepam	115	0	—	—	
Diazepam	115	0	—	—	
Lorazepam	115	4	31–49 pg/mg	40 pg/mg	22
Flunitrazepam	115	31	19–148 pg/mg	69 pg/mg	
Alprazolam	115	2	0.30–1.24 ng/mg	0.77 ng/mg	
Triazolam	115	0	—	—	
Nordiazepam	21	20	0.1–1.8 ng/mg	0.49 ng/mg	
Oxazepam	21	15	0.02–3.4 ng/mg	1.71 ng/mg	
Lormetazepam	21	3	4.1–29.1 ng/mg	17.09 ng/mg	23
Lorazepam	21	1	4.9 ng/mg	—	
Diazepam	21	15	0.01–2.2 ng/mg	0.31 ng/mg	
7-Amino-flunitrazepam	21	8	0.02–9.5 ng/mg	2.02 ng/mg	
Flunitrazepam	4	4	ND–23.00 pg/mg	12.38 pg/mg	24
7-Amino-flunitrazepam	4	4	ND–48.60 pg/mg	37.35 pg/mg	

[a]Concentrations before and after bleaching.

others were generally in the picogram per milligram range (flunitrazepam, 7-amino-flunitrazepam, lorazepam).

7. DETECTION OF FLUNITRAZEPAM AND 7-AMINO-FLUNITRAZEPAM

The procedure given here is used routinely at the Institute of Forensic Medicine of Strasbourg, France.

Before analysis, the hair sample is twice decontaminated in 5 mL of methylene chloride for 2 min at room temperature and pulverized in a Retsch MM2-type ball mill.

Fifty micrograms of powdered hair are incubated in 1 mL of Soerensen phosphate buffer, pH 7.6, overnight, at 40°C, in the presence of deuterated analogs (-d_3) of flunitrazepam and 7-amino-flunitrazepam (10 ng) used as internal standards. The homogenate is directly extracted with 5 mL of diethyl ether–chloroform (80:20, v/v). After horizontal agitation (20 min at 100 cycles/min) and centrifugation (15 min at 4000 rpm), the organic phase is removed and evaporated to dryness in a SpeedVac Concentrator (Savant A290). The residue is derivatized using 150 µL heptafluorobutyric anhydride–ethyl acetate (2:1, v/v), for 30 min at 60°C. The derivatized extract is reevaporated to dryness and dissolved in 25 µL of ethyl acetate before injection.

A 1.5-µL portion of the derivatized extract is injected on the column of a Hewlett Packard (HP) 5890 gas chromatograph, via a HP 7673 autosampler. The flow of carrier gas (helium, purity grade N55) through the column (HP-5MS capillary column, 5% phenyl–95% methylsiloxane, 30 m × 0.25 mm internal diameter) is 1.0 mL/min. The injector temperature is 240°C and splitless injection is employed with a split-valve off-time of 1.0 min. The temperature column is programmed to rise from an initial temperature of 60°C, kept for 1 min, to 295°C at 30°C/min and kept at 295°C for the final 6 min.

The detector used is a HP 5989 B Engine operating in NCI mode. The ion source and quadrupole temperature are 200°C and 100°C, respectively. The electron multiplier voltage is set at +400 V above the NCI-tune voltage. Methane is used as gas reactant at an apparent pressure of 1.3 torr in the ion source. Mass spectra are recorded in single-ion monitoring (SIM) mode.

Under the chromatographic conditions used, there is no interference with the drugs by any extractable endogenous materials present in hair. The ions chosen for quantification were the base peaks at *m/z* 313 for flunitrazepam-HFB (d_3: *m/z* 316) and *m/z* 459 for 7-amino-flunitrazepam-HFB (d_3: *m/z* 462).

Figure 1 show a typical SIM chromatogram of a hair specimen positive for flunitrazepam and its major metabolite, 7-amino-flunitrazepam. The concentrations were 391 and 823 pg/mg, respectively.

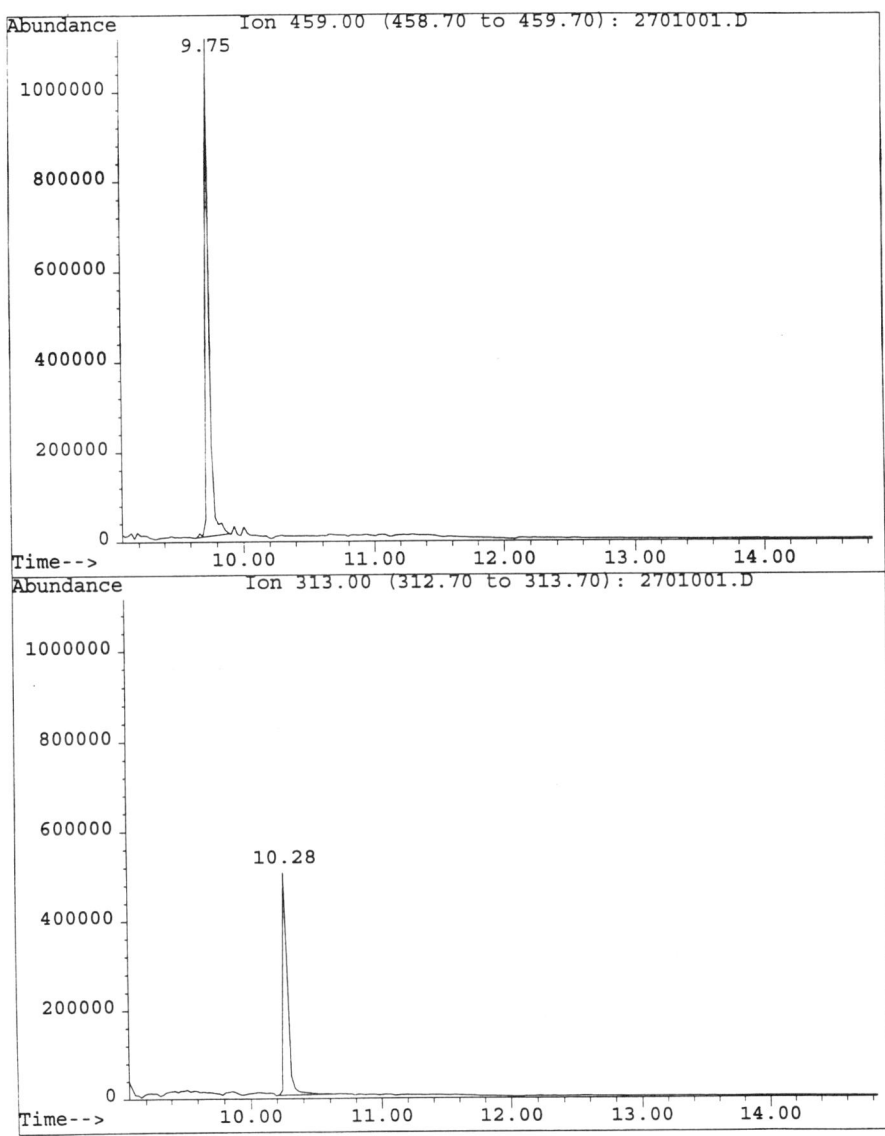

Fig 1. Typical SIM chromatogram of a hair specimen positive for flunitrazepam (m/z 313) and its major metabolite, 7-amino-flunitrazepam (m/z 459). Parent concentration was 391 pg/mg and 823 pg/mg for amino-flunitrazepam.

8. Conclusions

It appears that the value of hair analysis for the identification of drug users is steadily gaining recognition. This can be seen from its growing use in pre-employment screening, in forensic sciences, and in clinical applications. Hair analysis may be useful adjunct to conventional drug testing in toxicology. Specimens can be more easily obtained with less embarrassment, and hair can provide a more accurate history of drug use.

International conferences on hair analysis in Genoa (1994, 1996), Abu Dhabi (1995), Strasbourg (1997), Martigny (1999), and Kreicha (2000) indicate the increasing role of this method for the investigation on drug abuses.

Although GC/MS is the method of choice in practice, GC/MS/MS or liquid chromatography (LC)/MS are today used in several laboratories, even for routine cases, particularly to target low dosage compounds, such as flunitrazepam.

Today, quality assurance is a major issue of drug testing in hair. Since 1990, the National Institute of Standards and Technology (Gaithersburg, MD, United States) has developped inter-laboratory comparisons, recently followed by the new Society of Hair Testing (Strasbourg, France).

References

1. Baumgartner, W. A., Hill, V. A., and Blahd, W. H. (1989) Hair analysis for drugs of abuse. *J. Forensic Sci.* **34,** 1433–1453.
2. Negrusz, A. (2000) Single flunitrazepam abuse can be revealed by hair analysis! *ToxTalk* **24,** 4.
3. Harkey, M. R. and Henderson, G. L. (1989) *Advances in Analytical Toxicology* (Baselt, R. C., ed.), Year Book Medical Chicago, pp. 298–329.
4. Mangin, P. (1996) Drug analyses in nonhead hair, in *Drug Testing in Hair* (Kintz, P. ed.), CRC Press, Boca Raton, FL, pp. 279–288.
5. Yegles, M., Marson, Y., and Wennig R. (2000) Influence of bleaching on stability of benzodiazepines in hair. *Forensic Sci. Int.* **107,** 87–92.
6. Kintz, P. and Mangin, P. (1991) L'analyse des médicaments et des stupéfiants dans les cheveux—Intérêt et limites pour le diagnostique clinique et la toxicologie médico-légale. *J. Méd. Strasbourg* **22,** 518–522.
7. Sramek, J. J., Baumgartner, W. A., Ahrens, T. N., Hill, V. A., and Cutler, N. R. (1992) Detection of benzodiazepines in human hair by radioimmunoassay. *Ann. Pharmacother.* **26,** 469–472.
8. Kintz, P., Tracqui, A., and Mangin, P. (1992) Toxicological investigations on unusual materials (hair and vitreous humor): interest and limitations. *Arch. Toxicol.* **15,** 282–285.
9. Kintz, P., Tracqui, A., and Mangin, P. (1992) Detection of drugs in human hair for clinical and forensic. *Int. J. Legal Med.* **105,** 1–4.

10. Kintz, P., Ludes, B., and Mangin P. (1992) Detection of drugs in human hair using Abbott ADx with confirmation by gas chromatography/mass spectrometry (GC/MS). *J. Forensic Sci.* **37,** 328–331.
11. Kintz, P., Tracqui, A., and Mangin, P. (1992) Tabac, médicaments et stupéfiants pendant la grossesse—évaluation de l'exposition in utero par analyse des cheveux du nouveau-né. *Presse Méd.* **21,** 2139.
12. Kintz, P. and Mangin, P. (1993) Determination of gestational opiate, nicotine, benzodiazepines, cocaine and amphetamine exposure by hair analysis. *J. Forensic Sci.* **33,** 139–142.
13. Skopp, G. and Aderjan, R. (1993) Comparison of RIA and KIMS-immunoassay as tools for the detection of drug abuse patterns in human hair, in *Proceedings of the 31th International Meeting TIAFT* (Müller, R. K., ed.), Molinapress, Leipzig, pp. 446.
14. Kintz, P. and Mangin, P. (1995) Expertises judiciaires à partir d'échantillons de cheveux. *J. Méd. Lég. Droit Médic.* **38,** 241–244.
15. Kintz, P., Cirimele, V., and Mangin, P. (1995) Hair analysis for nordiazepam and oxazepam by gas chromatography-negative-ion chemical ionization mass spectrometry. *J. Chromatogr. B* **677,** 241–244.
16. Couper, F. J., Hons, B. Sc., McIntyre, I. M., and Drummer, O. H. (1995) Extraction of psychotropic drugs from human scalp hair. *J. Forensic Sci.* **40,** 83–86.
17. Segura, J. (1995) Possibilities of ELISA methodologies for hair analysis, in *Proceedings of the 1995 International Conference and Workshop for Hair Analysis in Forensic Toxicology*, 19–23 November 1995, Abu Dhabi, United Arab Emirates, pp. 350–369.
18. Cirimele, V., Kintz, P., and Mangin P. (1996) Detection and quantification of lorazepam in human hair by GC-MS/NCI in a case of traffic accident. *Int. J. Legal Med.* **108,** 265–267.
19. Cirimele, V., Kintz, P., and Mangin, P. (1996) Determination of chronic flunitrazepam abuse by hair analysis using GC/MS-NCI. *J. Analyt. Toxicol.* **20,** 596–598.
20. Gaillard, Y. and Pépin, G. (1996) Applications médico-légales de l'analyse des xénobiotiques dans les cheveux. *Toxicorama* **8,** 29–39.
21. Cirimele, V., Kintz, P., and Mangin, P. (1997) Testing human hair for flunitrazepam and 7-amino-flunitrazepam by GC/MS-NCI. *Forensic Sci. Int.* **84,** 189–200.
22. Cirimele, V., Kintz, P., and Ludes, B. (1997) Screening for forensically relevant benzodiazepines in human hair by gas chromatography-negative ion chemical ionization-mass spectrometry. *J. Chromatogr. B* **700,** 119–129.
23. Yegles, M., Mersch, F., and Wennig, R. (1997) Detection of benzodiazepines and other psychotropic drugs in human hair by GC/MS. *Forensic Sci. Int.* **84,** 211–218.
24. Negrusz, A., Moore, C., Deitermann, D., Lewis, D., Kaleciak, K., Kronstrand, R., et al. (1999) Highly sensitive micro-plate enzyme immunoassay screening and NCI-GC-MS confirmation of flunitrazepam and its major metabolite 7-amino-flunitrazepam in hair. *J. Analyt. Toxicol.* **23,** 429–435.

Chapter 6

γ-Hydroxybutyric Acid and Its Analogs, γ-Butyrolactone and 1,4-Butanediol

Laureen J. Marinetti

1. HISTORY AND PHARMACOLOGY OF GHB

Gamma-hydroxybutyric acid (GHB) is an endogenous compound in mammalian central nervous system and peripheral tissues and a minor metabolite or precursor of gamma-aminobutyric acid (GABA), an inhibitory neurotransmitter (Fig. 1). It was first synthesized in 1960 by Laborit *(1)* and his associates as an experimental GABA analog for possible use in the treatment of seizure disorder. They hypothesized that since GHB could readily cross the blood/brain barrier perhaps it could facilitate the synthesis of GABA in the brain. Although GHB did not produce elevated GABA synthesis, the research revealed that GHB had some pharmacologic properties that rendered it useful as an anesthetic adjuvant. The earliest pharmacological use of GHB in humans was in this application. Blumenfeld et al. *(2)* listed nine qualities observed from their experiments with GHB used in human anesthesia: mimics natural sleep, causes negligible reduction in minute respiratory volume, has cardiotonic effects, produces relaxation for ease of intubation, potentiates other central nervous system (CNS) depressants, does not change oxygen consumption, permits easy control of respiration, provides very stable vital signs, and permits slow induction of anesthesia. In this context Helrich et al. *(3)* correlated blood concentrations of GHB with state of consciousness in 16 adult human patients (Table 1).

From: *Forensic Science: Benzodiazepines and GHB: Detection and Pharmacology*
Edited by: S. J. Salamone © Humana Press Inc., Totowa, NJ

Fig. 1. Structures of GABA and GHB.

Table 1
Correlation of Blood Concentrations of GHB with State of Consciousness

	Sleep State			
	Awake	Light sleep	Medium sleep	Deep sleep
GHB (µg/mL)[a]	0–99	63–265	151–293	244–395

[a]Values converted from micromoles/per liter.

This study revealed that GHB blood concentrations as high as 99 µg/mL could be achieved with the patient still displaying an "awake" state. A light sleep state was characterized by the subject spontaneously coming in and out of consciousness. Subjects in the medium sleep state were clearly asleep but were able to be roused. At the highest concentrations studied GHB produced a deep sleep characterized by response to stimuli with a reflex movement only. It is clear from these data that blood concentrations of GHB display a large over-lap across the four states of consciousness described. For example, a subject with a blood concentration of 250 µg/mL could be in a light, medium, or deep sleep state. The smallest dose given, 50 mg/kg, produced peak plasma concentrations no greater than 182 µg/mL and the largest dose given, 165 mg/kg, produced peak plasma concentrations >416 µg/mL. Fourteen patients received doses of 100 mg/kg resulting in peak blood concentrations ranging from 234 to 520 µg/mL. Twelve of the 16 patients required intubation at this level of anesthesia but this did not necessarily correlate to those patients that received the higher doses of GHB. For example, one patient who received a dose of 75 mg/kg required intubation while another patient who received a dose of 100 mg/kg did not require intubation. Metcalf et al. *(4)* observed electroencephalographical (EEG) changes in 20 humans given oral doses of GHB in the range of 35 to 63 mg/kg. The EEG pattern was similar to that seen in natural slow wave sleep. Profound coma was observed at approximately 30 to 40 min post dose in subjects given oral GHB doses >50 mg/kg.

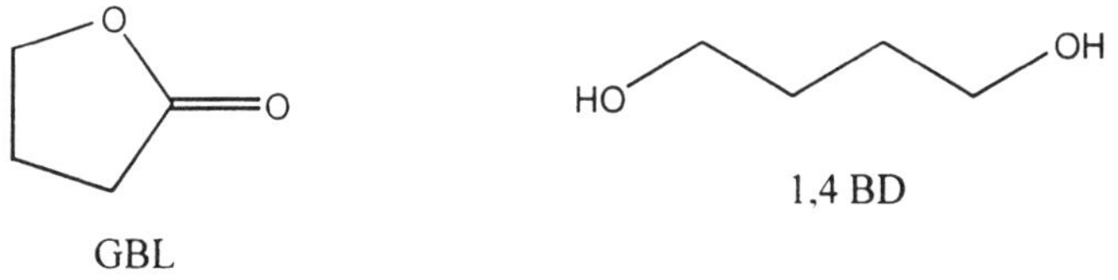

GHB and Its Analogs

Fig. 2. Structures of GBL and 1,4BD.

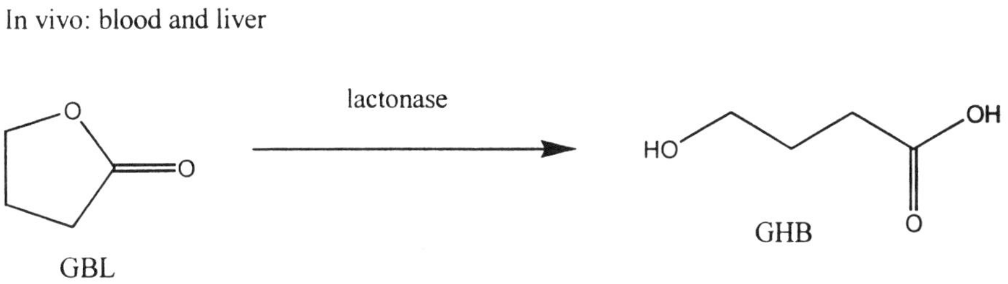

Fig. 3. A lactonase enzyme in blood and liver rapidly catalyzes the hydrolysis of GBL to GHB in vivo.

Research on GHB was expanded to include compounds that were analogs or metabolic precursors of GHB: γ-butyrolactone (GBL) and 1,4-butanediol (1,4BD) (Fig. 2). Sprince et al. *(5)* investigated the potential anesthetic properties of GBL and 1,4BD. Their observations that sleep induction time was the shortest with GBL and longest with 1,4BD as compared to GHB was an early clue to the metabolic relationship among these three compounds. Additional studies demonstrated that the pharmacologically active form of GBL was in fact GHB. Roth et al. *(6)* determined that when GBL and GHB were given by the intracisternal route GBL had no CNS depressant activity but an equal dose of GHB showed profound and lasting CNS depression. Roth and Giarman *(7)* determined that a lactonase enzyme in blood and liver rapidly catalyzed the hydrolysis of GBL to GHB (Fig. 3). Administration of the GHB and GBL intracisternally (i.e., directly into the CNS) provided no opportunity for biotransformation to occur, as the lactonase enzyme does not display any substantial activity in brain or cerebrospinal fluid (CSF). Several studies of GHB in the 1970s revealed that anesthetic doses of GHB cause an increase in dopamine concentration in the brain by blocking impulse flow in central dopaminergic neurons *(8–11)*. The net effect of blocking the impulse flow is to cause a buildup of dopamine in the dopaminergic nerve terminals because the synthesis of new dopamine continues while blocking the nerve impulse prevents dopamine release. Therefore, dopamine accumulates in the nerve terminal. Sethy et al. *(12)* determined that GHB may have a similar effect on brain concentration of acetylcholine, increasing acetylcholine concentration by decreasing impulse flow in cholinergic neurons. The reason GHB is abused is probably not attributable to an increase in concentration of brain dopamine by inhibition of its release *(13)*. Paradoxically at subanesthetic doses of GHB an excitation of dopamine neurons was observed *(14,15)*. Many drugs of abuse cause an increase in dopamine in the synapse via various mechanisms. Subanesthetic doses of GHB cause an initial stimulation of dopamine neurons, producing elevations of synaptic dopamine that may play a part in the reinforcing effect of GHB. Several researchers have demonstrated that GHB appears to have a distinct receptor site in the brain with both high and low affinity components. Current research suggests that this receptor appears to be a G-protein–coupled presynaptic receptor that is distinct from the $GABA_B$ receptor *(15a)*. In addition, there is also evidence that GHB is a weak agonist at the $GABA_B$ receptor *(16–20)*. However, the mechanism of action of GHB is still unresolved. Researchers have postulated that GHB has some capacity as a neurotransmitter and/or neuromodulator and investigation continues in this area.

2. HISTORY OF ILLICIT USE OF GHB

In 1977 a study was published that would permanently change the relative obscurity of GHB, GBL, and 1,4BD. Takahara et al. *(21)* administered GHB to six healthy adult males and showed an approx 10-fold increase in plasma growth hormone (GH) concentration that peaked at 45 min post dose. This effect persisted for about 15 min and then the GH concentration declined toward pretreatment level. GH concentration at 120 min post dose was still above baseline but significantly (2/3) below the peak concentration. Based on this report, bodybuilders assumed that they could increase GH concentration by using GHB and thereby optimize their muscle building potential. A more recent study by Van Cauter et al. *(22)* showed that the increase in GH secretion was correlated with the enhancement of slow wave sleep. GH release did not occur prior to sleep onset. The GH stimulating effect of a 2- to 3-g dose of GHB was seen during the first 2 h of sleep as an increase in amplitude and duration of the normal GH secretory pulse associated with sleep onset as opposed to an increase in the number of GH release pulses. A study by Addolorato et al. *(23)* on the effect on muscle mass of the GHB induced release of GH compared the muscle mass of patients on chronic GHB treatment for alcohol withdrawal syndrome to patients receiving psychological support alone. The researchers concluded that long-term administration of GHB did not affect muscle mass and were unable to detect an increase in GH release in the GHB treated group. A recent study has shown that the ability of GHB to increase GH in 4-yr abstinent alcoholics

Table 2
Product/Slang Names for GHB

Gamma OH	Scoop(s)
Sodium oxybate	Liquid ecstasy
Natural Sleep 500	Easy lay
Oxy-Sleep	Salt water
GHBA	Vita G
G-caps	Georgia home boy
G	Grevious bodily harm
Soap	Great Hormones at Bedtime
Liquid X	

does occur. The same subjects were evaluated for GH release by GHB at 2–3 wk of alcohol withdrawal and again after 4 year of abstinence, Vescovi and Coiro *(23a)*. At 2–3 wk of alcohol withdrawal the alcoholic subjects showed no increase in GH release with GHB administration. However after 4 years of abstinence these same alcoholic subjects did demonstrate an increase in GH release with GHB administration at nearly the same level as nonalcoholic subjects. It is hypothesized that this is due to a reconstitution over time of the neurotransmitter pathway underlying the GH releasing activity of GHB. It has been proposed by Volpi et al. *(23b)* that this is a muscarinic cholinergic pathway. In both the Vescovi and Coiro and the Volpi et al. studies it was not specifically mentioned whether the subjects were awake or asleep after GHB administration. In animal studies in both anesthetized and conscious rats and conscious dogs, various doses of GHB failed to increase GH concentration in any of the animals (Rigamonti and Müller; *23c*). The use of GHB by bodybuilders seemed harmless in theory until the emergency room reports started accumulating *(24)*.

Users soon discovered that GHB had a definite mood elevating quality and introduced GHB into the party drug scene, which is where it remains today in addition to its use as a natural health/diet aid. GHB is known by numerous street/slang names (Table 2). Most of these slang names utilize the letters G, H, B, such as "Georgia Home Boy" or Great Hormones at Bedtime. The slang name "liquid ecstasy" can be confusing, as "ecstasy" or XTC is the slang name commonly associated with methylenedioxymethamphetamine (MDMA), which is not in the same class of compounds as GHB. MDMA is a perception altering, entactogenic stimulant and is usually dispensed in pill form. In November of 1990 the FDA warned consumers of the danger of GHB, but the incidents of poisonings continued to rise. GHB and products containing GHB were removed from the market and GHB moved underground. Users soon discovered that GHB could easily be synthesized from readily available precursors. The industrial solvent, γ-butyrolactone, when made basic with lye and heated, would yield GHB. With addition of an acid such as vinegar to adjust the pH, the solution of GHB was ready to consume. This illicit GHB is especially dangerous because its concentration is unknown and can vary greatly from batch to batch. Also, contaminants may be introduced in the clandestine manufacturing process. GHB has a very steep dose–response curve so it is easy to accidentally overdose. Toxicity of GHB is characterized by euphoria, dizziness, visual disturbances, decreased level of consciousness, nausea, vomiting, suppression of the gag reflex, bradycardia, hypotension, acute delerium, confusion, agitation, hypothermia, random clonic muscle movements (twitching), coma, respiratory depression, and death. Although there have been some reports of seizures associated with GHB intoxication there is no evidence of true seizure activity as measured by EEG in humans *(25)*. However, only GHB doses consistent with safe anesthesia have been evaluated in these EEG studies. Clonic muscle movements and severe parasympathomimetic activity including profuse salivation, defecation, and urination have been documented in dogs treated with large doses (toxic and lethal) of GHB *(26)*. The muscle movement was so prominent at anesthetic doses that a barbiturate was also administered to effect convenient anesthesia. Perhaps some confusion exists between seizures and these clonic movements or muscle twitching. Another complicating factor is that GHB used outside a clinical setting is frequently used in combination with other drugs. This could affect the pharmacology of GHB in many ways depending on which additional drug(s) are consumed and their dose. By far the most common drug taken in combination with GHB is ethanol *(27–29)*. This combination is especially dangerous because ethanol potentiates GHB's CNS depressant effects as demonstrated by depression of the startle response (a measure of sensory responsiveness) in rats (Fig. 4) *(30)*. GHB has been implicated in fatalities both when administered alone *(31)* and when used in combination with other drug(s) *(32)*. The use of GHB has been implicated in drug-facilitated sexual assault. In fact, a common slang name for GHB is "date rape drug," although it is not deserving of this title. Actual confirmed cases in which GHB has been used in this capacity do exist but they are not common in comparison to other drugs more frequently chosen for this crime, namely ethanol and benzodiazepines. In a recent study analyzing urine specimens from alleged sexual assault victims, ethanol, cannabinoids, and benzodiazepines were the most common drugs detected *(33)*.

The most likely negative outcome of chronic GHB use is addiction. A GHB withdrawal syndrome has been documented with chronic GHB use *(34–*

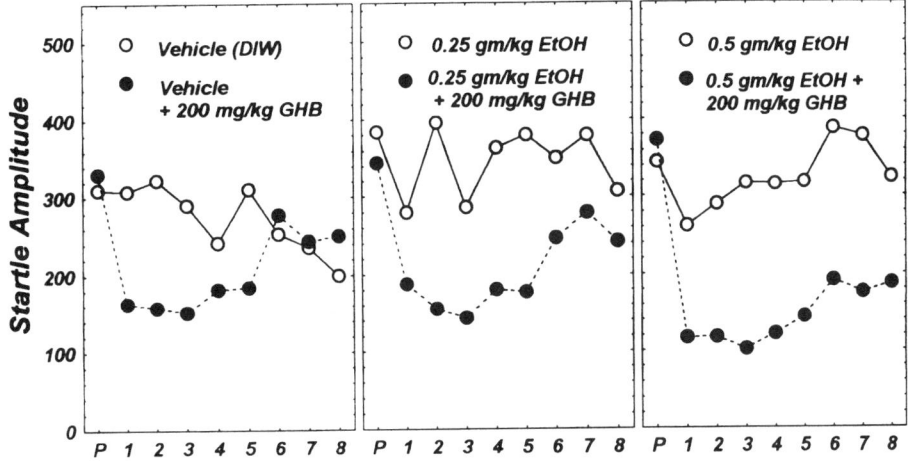

Time After Treatment (15-Min Intervals)

Fig. 4. Time course for the effects of 200 mg/kg GHB, administered alone or in combination with ethanol, on the acoustic startle response in the rat. Plotted are the mean values (n = 8–10 per point) for startle amplitude prior to drug treatment (P) and for various 15-min intervals following administration of vehicle (DIW, open circles) or 200 mg/kg GHB (filled circles) in rats coadministered vehicle (left panel), 0.25 gm/kg ethanol (middle panel); or 0.5 gm/kg ethanol (right panel). Neither ethanol dose administered alone affected startle amplitude compared to vehicle controls. GHB treatment reduced the startle amplitude; the magnitude and duration of this GHB-inducd reduction in startle amplitude was increased in subjects receiving ethanol cotreatment.

36). The clinical presentation of GHB withdrawal ranges from mild clinical anxiety, agitation, tremors, and insomnia to profound disorientation, increasing paranoia with auditory and visual hallucinations, tachycardia, elevated blood pressure, and extraocular motor impairment. Symptoms, which can be severe, generally resolve without sequelae after various withdrawal periods, although one documented death has occurred (36). Treatment with benzodiazepines has been successful for symptoms of a mild withdrawal syndrome.

3. CLINICAL USE OF GHB IN HUMANS

As discussed at the beginning of this chapter the first clinical uses of GHB were as an anesthetic adjuvant or induction agent. This application is still in use today in Europe (37). In the United States GHB is being evaluated primarily for the treatment of narcolepsy. A new drug application will likely

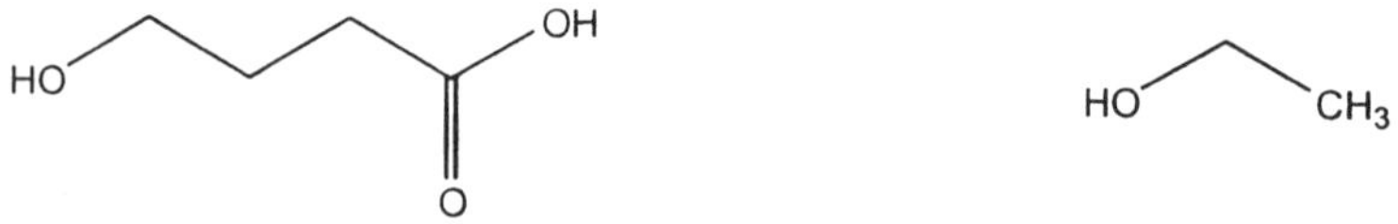

Fig. 5. Structures of GHB and ethanol.

be submitted to the FDA by the end of the year 2000 for sodium oxybate or Xyrem® (medically formulated GHB). Full approval is expected by the middle of the year 2001 *(38)*. At this time there is no medically approved use for GHB in the United States. Researchers feel that GHB will prove to be effective for the treatment of narcolepsy and its associated symptom, cataplexy, and will greatly improve the quality of life for suffers *(39,39a)*. This research has been ongoing since the 1970s and subjects participating in the clinical trails have experienced few adverse effects *(40)*. Another promising area for medically formulated GHB is in the treatment of alcohol withdrawal syndrome. This is not surprising since ethanol and GHB are similar compounds, both in structure and pharmacology (Fig. 5). Cross-tolerance between ethanol and subanesthetic doses of GHB has been observed in rats, which may explain why alcoholics being treated with GHB do not experience sedation at doses that would sedate a nonalcoholic individual *(40a)*. Exogenous administration of GHB has been shown to reduce ethanol consumption and intensity of ethanol withdrawal symptoms in rats and humans *(41–44)*. Adverse effects have been mild except for occasional replacement of alcohol addiction with GHB addiction, resulting in some subjects self-medicating with additional GHB to enhance its effects *(45)*. Treatment with GHB has also been investigated for opiate withdrawal syndrome *(46)*, cocaine addiction *(46a)*, and fibromyalgia *(47)*. For an in-depth review of GHB use in the treatment of withdrawal see the April 2000 volume 20, issue 3 of the journal *Alcohol*, where several articles are dedicated to this topic.

4. HISTORY OF ILLICIT USE OF *GBL* AND *1,4BD*

On February 18, 2000 GHB was placed in Federal Schedule I of the Controlled Substances Act, along with GBL, as a list I chemical as well as a controlled substance analog. 1,4BD was placed under the controlled substance analog section *(48,48a)*. This scheduling action included a provision for approved applications of medically formulated GHB, which will be placed in Federal Schedule III of the Controlled Substances Act.

Table 3
Chemical Synonyms for GBL

Dihydro-2(3H) furanone	4-Hydroxy-γ-lactone	4-Deoxytetronic acid
Butyrolactone-4	Butyrylactone	1,2-Butanolide
4-Butyrolactone	Butyrylactone	1,4-Butanolide
Butyric acid	γ-6480	4-Hydroxybutyric acid-γ-lactone
Butyric acid lactone	γ-BL	γ-Hydroxybutyric acid cyclic ester
Butyrolactone	BLO or BLON	NCI-C55875
α-Butyrolactone	4-Butanolide	Tetrahydro-2-furanone

Unfortunately, scheduling has not curbed the illicit use of this trio. There is more interest on the part of the illicit manufacturers in producing a GHB precusor product that will stay in the lactone form and not spontaneously convert to GHB because penalties for GBL are less severe. In fact, a seizure of solid GBL has recently been reported in California, where the liquid GBL was adsorbed onto silicon dioxide powder which was then placed into a clear capsule *(48b)*. This adds additional danger because the lactone form, based on its physical characteristics and its increased solubility in lipids, has been shown in animal studies to be absorbed by the gut more efficiently than the GHB acid. The FDA has requested removal of health supplement products containing GBL, but this is a small fraction of the products that contain this compound *(49)*. The most common use of GBL is as an industrial solvent with domestic production of approx 80,000 tons per year. In industry it is very widely used and would be difficult to replace based on its excellent properties as a safe, effective, and biodegradable degreaser. Some manufacturers of diet aid type products containing GBL have masked the presence of this ingredient by using one of the many chemical synonyms for GBL in the list of ingredients on the product label (Table 3).

Some products containing GBL include Renewtrient, Blue Nitro, and Invigorate. It has also been reported that GBL has been detected in alcoholic beverages, tobacco smoke, coffee, tomatoes, cooked meats, and several foodstuffs *(49a)*. The industrial solvent form of GBL is the product that is commonly used to illicitly manufacture GHB, as previously described. It has also been postulated that GBL could be illicitly manufactured from 1,4BD and tetrahydrofuran (THF). Although no source of illicit GBL from 1,4BD and THF has been identified, the synthesis is available on the Internet *(49b)*. GBL produces the same pharmacological effects as GHB as it is rapidly converted to GHB in the body. As mentioned previously, evidence in animal studies suggests that the lactone, being more lipophilic than GHB, is actually absorbed more readily. In fact GBL is considered the pro-drug for GHB and is commonly used in this capacity in animal studies *(50)*. At equimolar doses GBL produced a more prolonged hypnotic effect in rats as compared to GHB *(51)*. GBL has also been shown to produce cellular tolerance in mice *(51a,51b)*. To a lesser extent 1,4BD has followed the same path as GBL, although with the recent scheduling of GHB, 1,4BD is gaining in popularity and has recently been associated with adverse events including death *(51c,51d)*. An unconfirmed story from Russian folklore describes an ancient remedy for treating any sort of sexual dysfunction obtained from the oil of a small evergreen tree, the borametz tree *(52)*. Extracts of the borametz tree were commonly employed as an herbal remedy for sexual dysfuntion and more recently for increasing GH concentration. The tradition had very specific instructions regarding the proper use of the extract. Dosages were 1/2 to 2/3 of a teaspoon, taken on an empty stomach only at bedtime. Also borametz extract was not to be used at higher doses and it was never to be mixed with ethanol or other CNS depressants. When borametz extract was later analyzed by the Drug Enforcement Administration (DEA) it was found to contain 1,4BD. Hence some of the product names for 1,4BD; pine needle oil, herbal GHB, thunder nectar. This story was most likely created to promote the borametz oil product as the specific instructions with regard to CNS depressants and dose seem suspect; however, the borametz tree does exist and 1,4BD has been found in some plants. As with GBL, the major use for 1,4BD in the United States is as an industrial compound, with a projected usage in 2001 of 750,000,000 pounds. Unlike GBL however, 1,4BD is not used to illicitly manufacture GBL or GHB. This conversion is an industrial process and cannot be accomplished in a household setting. The pharmacological effects of 1,4BD are ultimately those of GHB, which is produced metabolically from 1,4BD in a two-step process (see Fig. 8). With the increased attention on GHB toxicity the FDA has also requested that products containing 1,4BD be removed from the market *(53)*. As with GBL this action could also lead manufacturers to replace the name, 1,4 butanediol, with one of its many chemical synonyms to disguise its presence in the product (Table 4).

5. METABOLISM OF GHB, GBL, AND 1,4BD

The predominant metabolic pathway for GHB is oxidation to succinc semialdehyde by a cytosolic $NADP^+$-dependent oxido-reductase enzyme called GHB dehydrogenase *(54,55)* (Fig. 6). This enzyme has been demonstrated in brain, liver, heart, spleen, testis, brown fat, and kidney, with liver, kidney, and brown fat having the greatest activity. An early study by Kaufman et al. concluded that GHB metabolism can also utilize NAD^+- depending on GHB

Table 4
Chemical Synonyms for 1,4BD

Butane-1,4-diol	Sucol B
1,4-Butylene glycol	1,4 Tetramethylene glycol
1,4-Dihydroxybutane	Butylene glycol
Diol 14B	Tetramethylene 1,4-diol

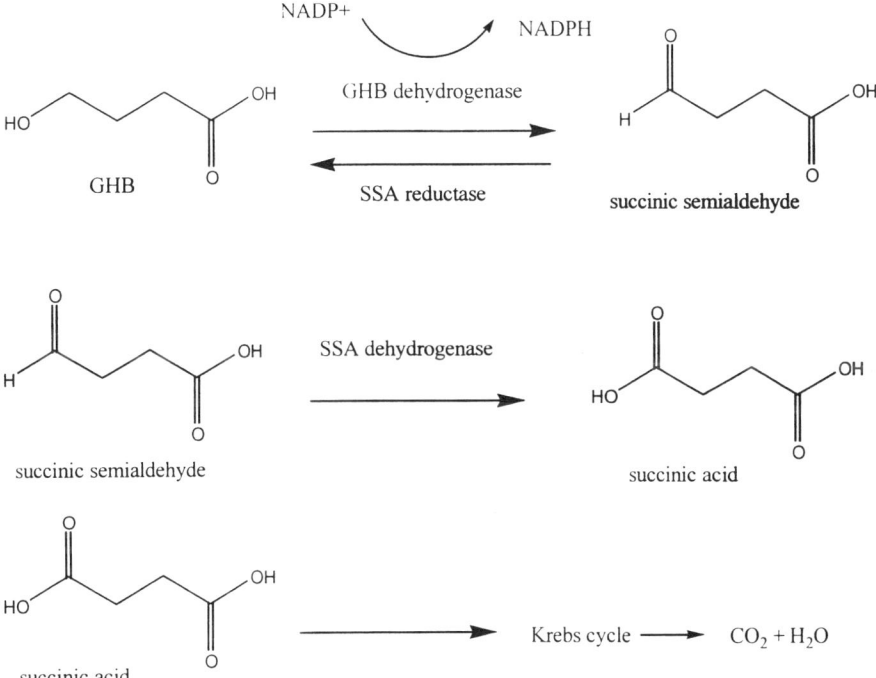

Fig. 6. The metabolism of GHB in vivo.

concentration and the tissue *(56)*. This study found that although liver has significant $NADP^+$ dependent GHB dehydrogenase activity, liver also has a large amount of NAD^+-dependent GHB dehydrogenase activity. In contrast, brain tissue exhibits exclusively $NADP^+$-dependent GHB dehydrogenase activity at lower GHB concentrations, with $NADP^+$ being the favored but not exclusive cofactor at higher GHB concentrations. The authors' observation that the utilization of NAD^+ in some circumstances of GHB metabolism is due to the fact that the second step of GHB metabolism involves an aldehyde type dehydrogenase enzyme, succinic semialdehyde dehydrogenase (see Fig. 6), which

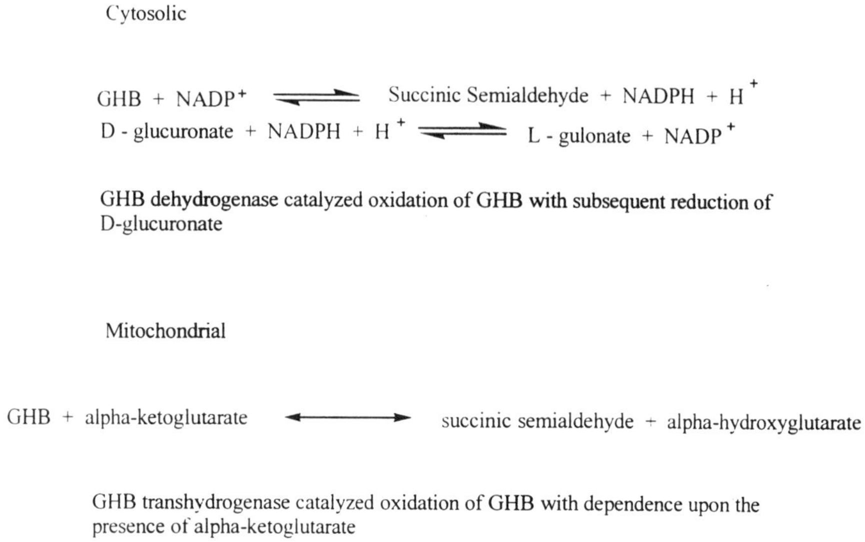

Cytosolic

GHB + NADP$^+$ ⇌ Succinic Semialdehyde + NADPH + H$^+$
D - glucuronate + NADPH + H$^+$ ⇌ L - gulonate + NADP$^+$

GHB dehydrogenase catalyzed oxidation of GHB with subsequent reduction of D-glucuronate

Mitochondrial

GHB + alpha-ketoglutarate ⇌ succinic semialdehyde + alpha-hydroxyglutarate

GHB transhydrogenase catalyzed oxidation of GHB with dependence upon the presence of alpha-ketoglutarate

Fig. 7. (a) GHB dehydrogenase catalyzed oxidation of GHB with subsequent reduction of D-glucuronate. (b) GHB transhydrogenase catalyzed oxidation of GHB with dependence upon the presence of α-ketoglutarate.

most likely utilizes NAD$^+$ as its cofactor just as the second step of ethanol metabolism uses aldehyde dehydrogenase to metabolize acetaldehyde to acetic acid with NAD$^+$ as the cofactor. Research to date does not indicate that alcohol dehydrogenase is capable of metabolizing GHB *(56–58)*. This could be an alternative pathway IF the normal pathway were to become saturated but no evidence exists to support this hypothesis. However, it has been suggested erroneously in some publications that alcohol dehydrogenase does normally metabolize GHB *(59)*. Kaufman and Nelson *(60)* have demonstrated that in addition to the required cofactor for GHB dehydrogenase activity, the enzyme is more efficient in vivo in a coupled reaction that involves subsequent D-glucuronate reduction to L-gulonate utilizing NADPH as the cofactor. These authors have also identified a second enzyme capable of oxidizing GHB to succinc semialdehyde. This enzyme is located in the microsomal fraction and requires no cofactor; however it is completely dependent on α-ketoglutarate in a coupled reaction. The enzyme, a hydroxyacid-oxoacid transhydrogenase named GHB transhydrogenase, can also catalyze the reverse reaction (Fig. 7). Some compounds formed in excess in natural disease states as well as some drugs have been demonstrated to inhibit GHB dehydrogenase. Drugs that have been found to inhibit GHB dehydrogenase include valproate, ethosuximide, salicylate, amobarbital, diphenylhydantoin, diethyldithiocarbamate (active form of disulfiram), and cyanide. It is not clear if therapeutic concentrations of these drugs would significantly inhibit GHB metabolism if the two were administered concurrently. A specific inhibitor of alcohol dehydrogenase, pyrazole, did not inhibit GHB dehydrogenase *(57)*. Various natural metabolic products that have been shown to inhibit GHB dehydrogenase include α-keto-isovalerate, α-keto-isocaproate, α-keto-β-methyl *n*-valerate (these three compounds are elevated in a condition called maple sugar urine disease), phenylacetate (elevated in persons with phenylketonuria [PKU]), and ketone bodies *(54)*. D-β-Hydroxybutyrate and acetoacetate, both ketone bodies, accumulate in persons with untreated diabetes or in a starvation state. In these abnormal conditions the elevated concentration of these naturally occurring metabolites could significantly inhibit the metabolism of GHB.

The second step in the metabolism of GHB is the oxidation of succinic semialdehyde to succinic acid via an NAD^+-dependent enzyme called succinic semialdehyde dehydrogenase. The succinic acid then becomes a substrate in the Krebs cycle and is ultimately metabolized to CO_2 and H_2O. A genetic disorder called GHB aciduria occurs when there is a deficiency of succinic semialdehyde dehydrogenase. Persons with this disorder have elevated concentrations of GHB in their blood, spinal fluid, and urine because excess succinic semialdehyde from GABA metabolism is reduced to GHB via succinic semialdehyde reductase, an NADPH dependent enzyme *(61)*. The clinical manifestations of the increased GHB concentration can range from mild oculomotor problems and ataxia to severe psychomotor retardation, but it is most commonly characterized by mental, motor, and language delay accompanied by hypotonia.

GBL is rapidly hydrolyzed to GHB in vivo with a half-life of less than 1 min. As previously stated, this reaction is catalyzed by an enzyme, lactonase, present in liver and blood. None of the other tissues and fluids that have been evaluated for lactonase activity, including brain, kidney, heart, lung, skeletal muscle, intestine, urine, and CSF, showed any substantial lactonase activity *(62)*. 1,4BD is also converted to GHB but not as rapidly as the GBL conversion. The conversion of 1,4BD to GHB requires two enzymatically catalyzed steps (Fig. 8). The first step is catalyzed by NAD^+- dependent alcohol dehydrogenase (ADH) *(63)*, producing γ-hydroxybutyraldehyde. The activity of ADH toward 1,4BD is similar to its activity towards ethanol and ethanol is a competitive inhibitor of 1,4BD metabolism to GHB. The second step is the conversion of γ-hydroxybutyraldehyde to GHB via a reaction catalyzed by aldehyde dehydrogenase. This aldehyde dehydrogenase mediated conversion can be inhibited by disulfiram. The liver, brain, kidney, and heart are able to convert

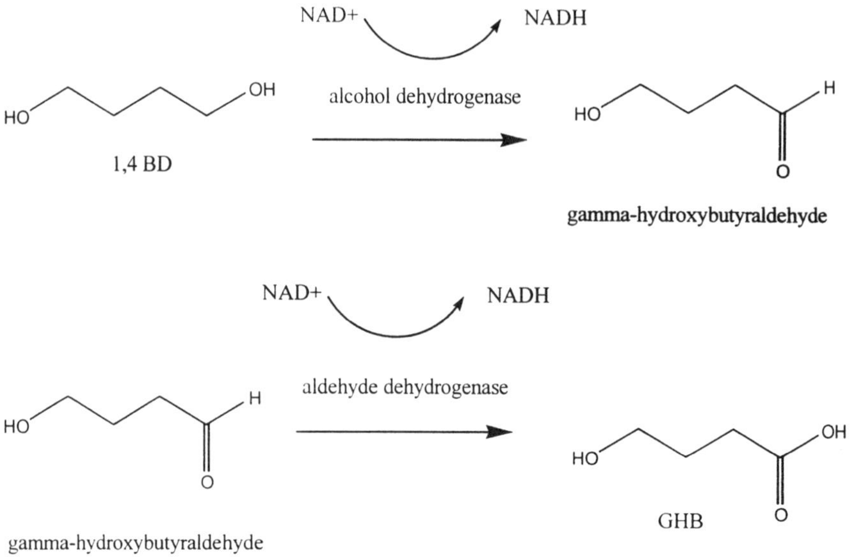

Fig. 8. The metabolism of 1,4BD to GHB in vivo.

1,4BD to GHB with the liver showing the greatest conversion capacity per gram of tissue *(63)*.

6. Distribution and Pharmacokinetics of GHB, GBL, and 1,4BD

Normal endogenous concentrations of GHB in CSF in humans are dependent on age and the presence of seizure disorder. Infants had higher concentrations of GHB (0.26–0.27 µg/mL) in the CSF than older children (0.11–0.13 µg/mL) who, in turn, had higher concentrations than adults (0.02–0.03 µg/mL). Children with myoclonic type seizures had the highest concentrations of GHB in the CSF (0.78–0.97 µg/mL), whereas children with other types of seizures had the next highest concentrations (0.37–0.48 µg/mL) *(64)*. Along with the analysis of the CSF for GHB the serum of all the subjects was also analyzed. Of the 130 subjects, none had any measurable amount of GHB in the serum, with a limit of sensitivity of the assay of 0.002 µg/mL. In another study GHB concentrations were determined in various tissues and blood of rats *(65)*. The results, converted from nanomoles per gram to microgram per gram or microgram per milliliter (blood), are given in Table 5.

Brown fat, kidney, muscle, and heart showed concentrations greater than 1 µg/g. Liver, lung, blood, brain, and white fat had concentrations lower than 0.25 µg/g. The reason for the variations in GHB content between the speci-

Table 5
Distribution of Endogenous GHB in Various Rat Specimens

	Brain	Heart	Kidney	Liver	Lung	Muscle	Blood	White fat	Brown fat
GHB range (µg/g)	0.14–0.24	0.63–1.6	1.5–3.0	0.08–0.25	0.07–0.17	0.83–1.5	0.03–0.08	0.02–0.07	3.7–4.1

mens analyzed is not known at this time. A study that compared endogenous GHB concentrations in brain from human, monkey, and guinea pig showed an elevated concentration as compared to that seen in rat brain, 0.2–2 µg/g, 0.3–1.8 µg/g, and 0.1–0.6 µg/g, respectively (66). In this same study endogenous GHB in CSF and blood of humans was found in only trace amounts (CSF ~0.01 µg/mL). The distribution of GHB into the CSF appears to lag behind that in blood or brain. After a 500 mg/kg intravenous dose of GHB was administered to dogs, plasma concentration peaked within 5 min, brain concentration peaked within 10 min, but it was 170 min before CSF concentrations reached their maximum (67). Snead et al. (67a) observed a similar distribution of GHB in serum and CSF in cats with time to peak CSF concentration lagging behind time to peak serum concentration by 40–100 min, depending on the initial dose, and at 60–120 min after GHB infusion CSF concentration exceeded serum concentration. This suggests a passive diffusion of GHB from serum or brain into the CSF. In alcohol dependent patients GHB did not accumulate in the body on repeated doses nor did it exhibit any protein binding. The mean peak plasma concentrations of therapeutic oral doses of 25 and 50 mg/kg of GHB per day given to 50 alcohol withdrawal syndrome patients were 55 µg/mL (range = 24–88) and 90 µg/mL (range = 51–158), respectively (68).

Absorption of GHB has been shown to be a capacity limited process with increases in dose resulting in increases in time to peak concentration. The concentration in brain equilibrates with other tissues after approximately 30 min. GHB crosses the placental barrier at a similar rate to that in the blood/brain barrier (69). GHB also exhibits first-pass metabolism when given orally with about 65% bioavailability when compared to an equivalent intravenous dose.

GHB exhibits zero-order (constant rate) elimination kinetics after an intravenous dose. Since GHB exhibits zero-order kinetics it has no true half-life. The time required to eliminate half of a given dose increases as the dose increases. A daily therapeutic dose of 25 mg/kg has an apparent half-life of about 30 min in humans as determined in alcohol dependent patients under GHB treatment (70). In contrast, an apparent half-life of 1–2 h was observed in dogs when they were given high intravenous doses of GHB. In humans it has been documented that there is increased rate of absorption if GHB is administered on an empty stomach resulting in a reduced time to reach maximum plasma concentration of GHB *(70a)*.

The absorption of GBL has been documented to occur faster than GHB. This occurs because the lactone form is much more lipophilic or nonpolar and can therefore cross cell membranes much more readily than GHB. For this reason GBL is often referred to as the pro-drug of GHB *(71)*. It has also been proposed that in addition to the better absorption of GBL it may also distribute differently than GHB. An early study comparing the distribution of equimolar doses of GHB and GBL in rats found that although peak plasma concentrations were higher with GHB they remained elevated longer with GBL. In addition, concentrations of GBL in the lean muscle mass of the rat were always elevated compared to concentrations of GHB *(62)*. This suggests sequestration of GBL into lean muscle prior to its conversion to GHB. Since lean muscle does not contain the lactonase enzyme, it is conceivable that this could occur. The GBL could then redistribute into the blood to be converted to GHB by the blood or liver lactonase enzyme. This could explain the prolonged elevated concentrations of GHB in blood that occur when GBL is given. Neither GHB nor GBL are sequestered in fat.

The absorption and distribution of 1,4BD is quite similar to GHB. It is a lipophobic or polar compound so it does not absorb faster than GHB. After its absorption it requires a two step enzymatic conversion to GHB that results in a slightly longer time to peak GHB concentration and also a longer time of elevated GHB concentration. As discussed previously, the conversion process of 1,4BD to GHB can be slowed or inhibited by ethanol, pyrazole, or disulfiram.

7. GHB INTERPRETATION ISSUES AND POSTMORTEM PRODUCTION

Animal and human studies have demonstrated that endogenous GHB concentrations can rise postmortem and under inappropriate specimen storage conditions. Doherty et al. *(66)* observed an increase in the GHB concentrations in brain specimens after 6 h with a further increase if the specimens were left at room temperature. Snead et al. *(64)* also observed an increase in GHB concentrations in CSF after 12 h of storage at room temperature. It was subsequently discovered that if animals were killed using microwave irradiation that postmortem GHB accumulation was blocked *(72)*. This suggests some type of enzymatic conversion from a GHB precursor. Succinic semialdehyde has been proposed as a possible source. This could occur by two pathways.

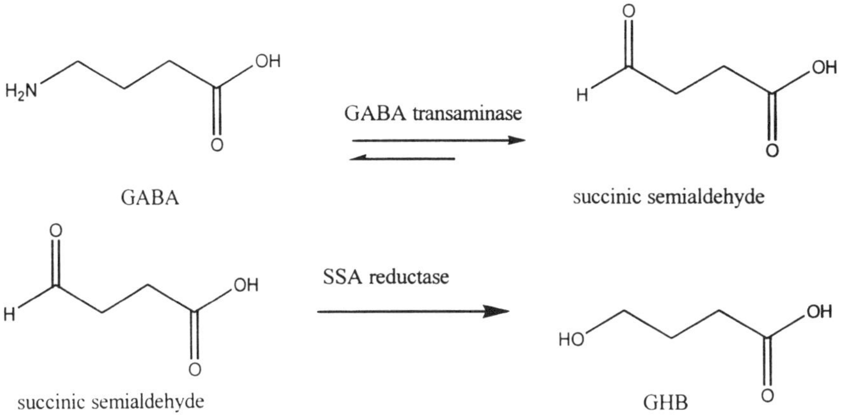

Fig. 9. GABA metabolism to GHB in vivo.

After death a cessation of Krebs cycle activity occurs which would result in an increase in substrates that normally would utilize this pathway, succinic acid being one. The buildup of succinic acid would drive the reaction toward succinic semialdehyde and succinic semialdehyde reductase would convert the succinic semialdehyde to GHB. The second pathway involves the metabolism of previously sequestered GABA that is being released from storage vesicles as the natural decomposition process occurs. Excess GABA would be exposed to the GABA transaminase enzyme which could convert it to succinic semialdehyde which could in turn be converted to GHB (Fig. 9) in addition to proceeding on to succinic acid (Fig. 10). However, the most likely source of postmortem GHB production is putrescine (1,4-butanediamine), a biogenic polyamine initially detected in decaying animal tissues, but now known to be present in all cells, both eukaryotic and prokaryotic, where it is important for cell proliferation and differentiation *(73)*. Research on polyamine metabolism by Seiler *(74)* demonstrated the formation of GABA from putrescine both in visceral organs and in the CNS of vertebrates. This is a two-step enzymatic process in the polyamine metabolic pathway that involves diamine oxidase (DAO) and aldehyde dehydrogenase to form GABA (Fig. 11). In organs that do not contain high activity of DAO, such as brain, an alternative pathway is available for the conversion of putrescine to GABA. This pathway involves the conversion of putrescine to monoacetylputrescine by the enzymatic addition via polyamine aminotransferase of acetyl CoA. Monoacetylputrescine is a substrate for monoamine oxidase (MAO). The subsequent action of MAO on monoacetylputrescine, then aldehyde dehydrogenase, followed by acetylpolyamine

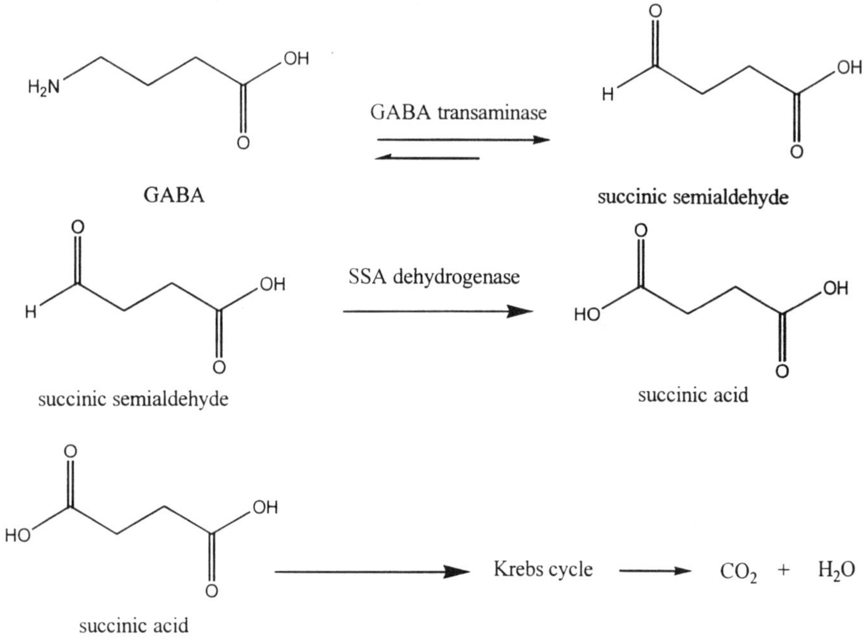

Fig. 10. GABA metabolism in vivo.

deacetylase, forms GABA (Sessa and Perin; *74a*). In addition Snead et al. *(75)* observed an 80–100% increase in GHB concentrations in rat brain after intracerebroventricular administration of putrescine. All of these theories are consistent with the observation that microwave irradiation prevents postmortem accumulation of GHB as the exposure to the microwaves would denature the enzymes. This is also supported by the fact that excessive GHB production is not seen in blood specimens that have an enzyme inhibitor added *(76)*. Regardless of the source of the increased concentration of GHB postmortem it can be a significant problem in determination of a cause of death due to GHB toxicity. Postmortem production of GHB can result in blood concentrations of GHB that would produce significant effects in a living person. Anderson and Kuwahara *(77)* analyzed heart blood, femoral blood, and urine from 96 postmortem cases with no suspected exogenous GHB use and from 50 antemortem blood specimens also with no evidence of GHB use. The specimens were stored at 4°C with sodium fluoride added to the blood as a preservative. They obtained the following results in the postmortem specimens: heart blood, 1.6–36 µg/mL; femoral blood, 1.7–48 µg/mL; and urine, 0–14 µg/mL, and no detectable amount of GHB in any of the antemortem blood specimens, with a limit of detection of 0.5 µg/mL. The upper end of the postmortem blood range over-

GHB and Its Analogs

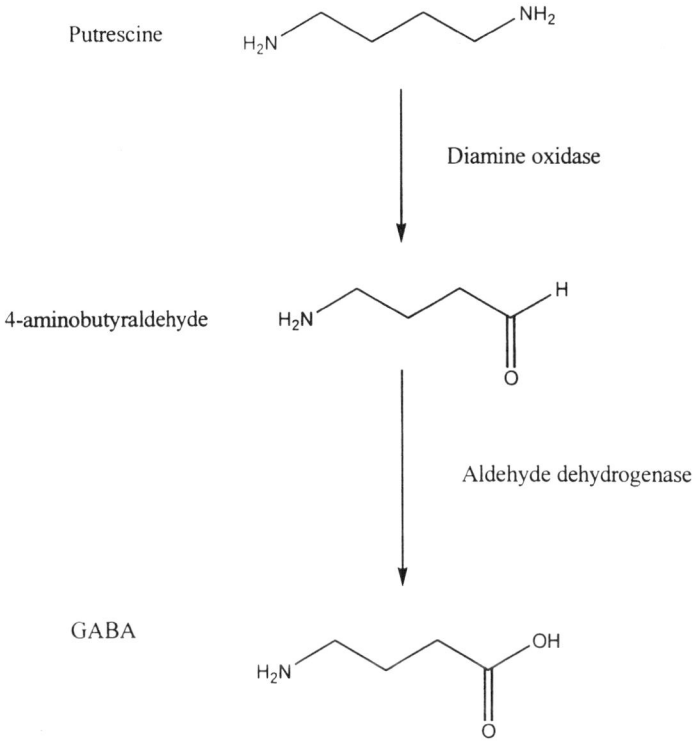

Fig. 11. Formation of GABA from putrescine in polyamine metabolism.

laps the range detected in blood during therapeutic application of a 25 mg/kg per day dose of GHB, 24–88 µg/mL. If one compares this to the highest concentrations that were discussed earlier in antemortem blood and CSF, 1 µg/mL in the CSF of children with myoclonic type seizure disorder, it is obvious that these are significant concentrations. Also the fact that there is very little difference between GHB concentrations in heart and femoral blood suggests that this is not simply a postmortem redistribution issue. In a similar study by Fieler et al. *(78)* a range of 0–168 µg/mL (average 25 µg/mL) in postmortem blood was observed with no detectable GHB in postmortem urine or antemortem blood or urine, with a limit of detection of 1 µg/mL. Although these data showed a larger concentration range than the data of Anderson et al., an average of 25 µg/mL for 20 blood specimens indicates that the majority of the concentrations were at the lower end of the range. The Fieler et al. study does not discuss the storage conditions of the specimens prior to analysis, which has been shown to have an effect on the amount of postmortem GHB produced. Stephens et al. *(76)* compared postmortem GHB concentrations in samples under various storage conditions. They found that GHB concentrations increased by 50% if the specimen did not contain sodium fluoride even when it was stored in a refrigerator, and if the specimen was stored at room temperature without 10 mg/mL sodium fluoride the concentration could double. The addition of sodium fluoride did not affect the concentration of GHB in urine specimens that were compared. Antemortem blood preserved with citrate (yellow top tube) has been shown to display an increase in GHB concentration over time (LeBeau et al.; *78a*). Ten antemortem-citrate-buffered whole blood specimens were analyzed for GHB after various storage periods from 6 to 36 mo at −20°C. Although no exogenous GHB use was suspected, all of the specimens had concentrations of GHB ranging from 4 to 13 µg/mL, with a mean of 9 µg/mL. The real problem this presents is in the interpretation of exogenous GHB use, GHB toxicity, or GHB overdose resulting in a fatality. Since GHB is rapidly cleared from the body, even at elevated doses, if there is any survival time the blood concentrations can easily fall into the range of postmortem production. Therefore, a urine specimen should be collected in addition to blood in suspected GHB cases. If urine is not available, then eye fluid or CSF is indicated, especially CSF because the normal endogenous concentration of GHB in CSF is well documented. It is advisable to preserve all specimens with at least 10 mg/mL sodium fluoride and store at refrigerator temperature or freeze and to avoid citrate-containing tubes. At this time there are no published data on endogenous GHB concentrations in postmortem eye fluid and certainly none for antemortem eye fluid. Organ specimens may also be helpful, but again there are no published data on endogenous concentrations of GHB in various organs in humans. The cutoff concentration for reporting exogenous GHB consumption in a specimen must be set above the suspected postmortem production or antemortem endogenous GHB concentration. This is not too difficult in the case of an antemortem specimen, provided it is not from a citrate-containing tube, but it can be very difficult in certain postmortem specimens.

Data from analyses of multiple specimens and a good case history can help tremendously especially if litigation is involved. For example, in a case that involved the death of a young girl and GHB, a postmortem blood GHB concentration of 15 µg/mL was demonstrated. This concentration is in the range of postmortem GHB production. However, a detailed case history plus a postmortem urine GHB concentration of 150 µg/mL, an antemortem blood concentration of 510 µg/mL, an antemortem urine concentration of 2300 µg/mL, and the lack of any other significant autopsy findings made the cause of death an obvious GHB fatality. The deceased had a 14 h survival time in the hospital prior to death, which explains the low postmortem blood GHB concentration *(31)*. A second GHB fatality showed a heart blood concentration of 66 µg/mL,

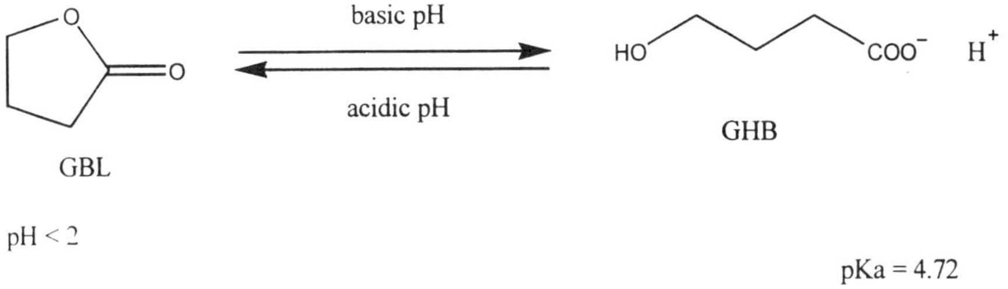

Fig. 12. The dynamic equilibrium of GHB and GBL in vitro or in the absence of the lactonase enzyme in vivo.

a femoral blood concentration of 77 μg/mL, an eye fluid concentration of 85 μg/mL, and a urine concentration of 1260 μg/mL. This individual had an extensive history of chronic GHB use and no other cause of death *(31)*. In this author's experience, two other cases demonstrated postmortem GHB concentrations of 310 μg/mL in blood with a urine concentration of 2100 μg/mL and in the second case a concentration of 410 μg/mL in blood with an eye fluid concentration of 212 μg/mL. These concentrations indicate a much more acute intoxication with little survival time and are consistent with GHB concentrations seen in deep anesthesia.

8. ANALYSIS FOR *GHB, GBL,* AND *1,4BD*

GHB does not exist in a static state, even outside of the body. In solution, it exists in a dynamic state in equilibrium with its lactone, GBL (Fig. 12). The ratio of the two forms is dependent on the pH of the matrix or the type of matrix containing the GHB. For example, in blood, the GHB acid form predominates because the lactonase enzyme converts any of the lactone to the acid. However if the GHB is in a matrix that does not contain this enzyme, such as urine, water, or juice, the two forms will reach equilibrium with both being present. The form that predominates depends on the pH of the solution, with lower pH favoring the lactone form, GBL. Complete conversion to GBL is favored in dehydrating conditions at pH below 2 in a concentrated acid solution. This can be achieved by the addition of a concentrated, dehydrating acid such as sulfuric acid. The rate at which the equilibrium is reached depends on the temperature and the actual pH of the matrix.

There are two basic approaches to GHB and GBL analysis depending on the matrix being analyzed. If a biological matrix is being analyzed, then conversion of GHB to GBL or derivatization of the GHB without conversion is acceptable, as a biological matrix should not normally contain any GBL with the exception of the stomach contents. However, it is possible that a urine specimen (or any other biological specimen that does not contain the lactonase enzyme) with a low pH (5 or 6) might produce GBL from GHB upon longterm storage. An excellent study that demonstrated this potential was done by Ciolino and Mesmer *(79)*. The authors compared solutions of GHB and GBL in various matrices at various pH values and found that the relative amounts of GHB and GBL changed depending on the pH of the matrix and storage conditions, specifically time and temperature. Anderson et al. reported a fatality that displayed measurable concentrations of GBL in heart and femoral blood, vitreous humor, liver, bile, gastric contents, and urine *(79a)*. Perhaps this is evidence of a massive GBL ingestion that resulted in saturation of the lactonase enzyme since the concentrations of GHB in this case were very high, with a heart blood concentration of 1,473 µg/mL. However, if 1,4BD is ingested, because it is not in equilibrium with GHB or GBL, unchanged 1,4BD may be detected in a biological specimen if enough is ingested and/or the time interval since ingestion is short *(80)*. Analyses of illicit or commercial products to determine GHB or GBL require that either two aliquots of sample be analyzed if the GHB to GBL conversion is used, or that a derivatization method be used so that the percentage composition of GHB in the sample can be determined. Knowing the actual percentage of GHB and GBL in the sample may be important in the documentation of a product source in both criminal and civil litigation cases.

Biological specimen extraction can be accomplished by liquid/liquid, solid phase, or solid phase microextraction with subsequent detection of GHB or GBL by gas chromatography/mass spectrometry (GC/MS) using electron impact (EI), positive or negative chemical impact (CI), or gas chromatography with flame ionization detection (GC/FID). LeBeau et al. *(81)* describe a method that employs two aliquots of specimen. The first is converted to GBL with concentrated sulfuric acid while the second is extracted without conversion. A simple liquid/liquid methylene chloride extraction was employed, and the aliquots were then screened by GC/FID without derivatization. Specimens that screened positive by this method were then aliquoted again and subjected to the same extraction with the addition of the deuterated analogs of GHB and GBL. These extracts were then analyzed by headspace GC/MS in the full-scan mode. Quantitation was performed by comparison of the area of the molecular ion of the parent drug (m/z 86) to that of the deuterated analog (m/z 92). This method displayed linearity in both blood and urine from 5 to 1000 µg/mL with recoveries that averaged between 75% and 87%. A liquid/liquid extraction method employed by the toxicology laboratory in the Department of the Coroner of Los Angeles County California *(82)* first converts GHB to the lactone followed by chloroform extraction. Both blood and urine were analyzed using this method with γ-valerolactone as the internal standard. Detection was by GC/MS using selected ion monitoring (SIM) mode. The following ions are monitored: GBL 42, 56, and 86 with 41, 56, and 85 for the internal standard. The method was linear from 5 to 300 µg/mL, with a lower limit of detection of 5 µg/mL. Couper and Logan *(83)* describe a liquid/liquid extraction method that uses ethyl acetate to extract GHB, without conversion to GBL. The extract is derivatized using *N,O-bis*-(trimethylsilyl)trifluoroacetamide (BSTFA) with 1% trimethylchlorosilane (TMCS) and acetonitrile and then analyzed using GC/MS in EI mode with selected ion monitoring of m/z 233, 204, and 117 for GHB and m/z 235, 103, and 117 for the diethylene glycol internal standard. The method gave a 55% extraction recovery of GHB in blood, with a limit of detection in blood and urine of 0.5 µg/mL, and a linearity of 1 to 100 µg/mL in blood and 1 to 200 µg/mL in urine. Another liquid/liquid extraction which is very similar to Couper and Logan's method has been described by Elian *(84)*. The differences between this method and the Couper and Logan method are its use of d_6-GHB as the internal standard, its evaluation only of urine specimens, and its 80 to 85% recovery, with linearity from 2 to 50 µg/mL.

There are three different solid phase extraction (SPE) methods that differ with respect to the column used, preextraction sample treatment, postextraction sample treatment, and internal standard. All three SPE methods extract GHB from urine and blood, derivatize with BSTFA with 1% TMCS and detect analytes by GC/MS in the EI mode either with SIM or full scan. The ions monitored for the GHB di-TMS derivative are 233, 234, and 235 with care being taken to avoid the ions that are common between di-TMS GHB and di-TMS urea, 147, 148, and 149. Urea is a naturally occurring compound in urine and care must be taken so that its derivative does not interfere. The SPE method used by the Miami-Dade County Medical Examiner's Office, Toxicology Laboratory in Miami, Florida *(85)* uses Chem-Elute® SPE columns, β-hydroxybutyric acid internal standard, pretreatment of urine with sulfuric acid, and pretreatment of blood with sodium tungstate and sulfuric acid. The Dade County method gave an absolute recovery of 30%, with a limit of detection of 2 µg/mL and a limit of quantitation of 10 µg/mL. McCusker et al. *(86)* describe a method for urine that uses United Chemical Technologies® GHB SPE column. Urine, GHB-d_6 internal standard, and phosphate buffer are combined and extracted. The final eluent is taken to dryness and then reconstituted with hexane and dimethylformamide (DMF). After a simple liquid/liquid extraction the hexane layer is discarded, the DMF is taken to dryness, and the residue is derivatized with BSTFA with 1%TMCS in ethyl acetate. The method gave a linearity range from 5 to 500 µg/mL. The limit of sensitivity or percent recovery of the method was not reported. The United Chemical Technologies® GHB SPE column method has been modified to include GHB and 1,4BD analysis in blood, eye fluid, and tissue homogenate samples. Sample size is only 200 µL and requires a sample preparation step of extraction with acetone prior to elution on the SPE column. The eluent from the SPE column, which is in 99/1 methanol/ammonium hydroxide, is then taken to dryness and derivatized with BSTFA with 1% TMCS. The ions monitored are 233, 234, and 235 for GHB di-TMS; 239, 240, and 241 for GHB-d_6 di-TMS; 219, 220, and 221 for 1,4BD di-TMS; and 223, 224, and 225 for 1,4BD-d_4 di-TMS *(51c,87)*. The third SPE method utilizes a Multi-Prep® Anion Exchange GVSA-200 Gravity Flow Column and is used for urine or blood analysis *(88)*. This is a very simple SPE procedure that involves mixing the specimen with pH 9 Tris buffer prior to extraction and passing all solutions through the column by gravity flow. This investigational method utilized GHB-d_6 as the internal standard and displayed linearity from 1 to 500 µg/mL with a recovery greater than 90%. A GC/MS method with negative ion detection is described for the measurement of GHB in rat brain *(89)*. It involves a complicated liquid/liquid extraction with subsequent derivatization of GHB with MTBSTFA. This method is very sensitive with the capability of detecting as little as 2 pg of neat GHB. The standard curve ranged from 0 to 64 ng of GHB. Measurement of endogenous antemortem concentration of GHB would be an appropriate application for this method, but forensic analysis of biological specimens for GHB does not require limits of detection this low. Frison et al. *(90)* describe a method using solid phase microextraction of GHB in plasma and urine. This is a new approach for GHB analysis that shows promise in that it is simple, sensitive, and requires only 0.5 mL of specimen. The linearity range was 1–100 µg/mL in plasma and 5 to 150 µg/mL in urine, with a limit of detection of 0.05 µg/mL and 0.1 µg/mL for plasma and urine respectively. The limit of detection was calculated based on aqueous solutions because the blank plasma and urine specimens had endogenous GHB concentrations of 0.1–0.2 µg/mL and 0.5–1.5 µg/mL, respectively. Therefore, it is important to evaluate the possibility of significant GHB concentrations in blank matrices prior to their use. The method required conversion of GHB to GBL with d_6-GBL as the internal standard and detection by headspace GC/MS with spectra from both CI and EI ionization modes. Many methods are available for GHB and GBL analyses depending on the equipment and resources available to the laboratory.

However, the same is not true for 1,4BD analysis. Concern over detecting and quantifying 1,4BD is just becoming an issue in the forensic community. As discussed previously, the pharmacologically active form of 1,4BD is GHB. However, determination of the concentration of 1,4BD may be useful in documenting acute intoxication. McCutcheon et al. *(80)* utilizes a simple one-step extraction at physiological pH into *n*-butyl chloride for the extraction of 1,4BD. The solvent is dried down to about 75 µL and subjected to GC/MS analysis. The 1,4BD elutes prior to GBL, with a detection limit between 50 and 100 µg/mL. Research by the authors is currently underway to improve this method. A method specific for the dectection of 1,4BD in liver and brain tissue is described by Barker et al. *(91)*. This method involves a complicated extraction scheme that utilizes different extraction protocols for the aqueous and lipid fractions of the tissues. Both fractions are then lyophilized to dryness, extracted again, and subsequently derivatized with heptafluorobutyric anhydride (HFBA). The internal standard used was deuterated 1,4BD with identification and quantitation by electron impact GC/MS in the SIM mode. Both rat and human brain tissue were analyzed in addition to rat liver. The method demonstrated a recovery of 74% ± 10% for the aqueous fraction and 88% ± 9% for the lipid fraction. The linearity range was 0.0 to 1.0 µg/g wet weight of tissue, with a limit of detection of 0.01 µg/g wet weight of tissue. Also, as was mentioned previously, the United Chemical Technologies® GHB SPE column method has been modified to include 1,4BD analysis *(51c)*. This method is currently in use by this author for analysis of both GHB and 1,4BD.

In conclusion, despite of or because of its simple structure GHB is a complicated multifacted compound that continues to be an issue in forensic toxicology. In addition to prevalence of GBL and 1,4BD as industrial compounds and the availability of GBL and 1,4BD on the Internet (www.chemicalkits.com), the GHB issue is here to stay. Readers should continue to monitor the journals for new discoveries and relevations concerning GHB and its analogs that are sure to come. Finally, it should be noted that although this chapter focused on the English language database, there are hundreds of references in many other languages concerning GHB and its analogs that are not represented in this work.

References

1. Laborit, H., Jouany, J. M., Gerard, J., and Fabiani, F. (1960) Generalites concernant l'etude experimentale de l'emploi clinique du gamma hydroxybutyrate de Na. *Aggressologie* **1**, 407.
2. Blumenfeld, M., Suntay, R. G., and Harmel, M. H. (1962) Sodium gamma-hydroxybutyric acid: a new anesthetic adjuvant. *Anesth. Analges.* **41**, 721–726.
3. Helrich, M., McAslan, T. C., Skolnik, S., and Bessman, S. P. (1964) Correlation of blood levels of 4-hydroxybutyrate with state of consciousness. *Anesthesiology* **25**, 771–775.
4. Metcalf, D. R., Emde, R. N., and Stripe, J. T. (1966) An EEG-behavioral study of sodium hydroxybutyrate in humans. *Electroencephalogr. Clin. Neurophysiol.* **20**, 506–512.

5. Sprince, H., Josephs, J. A., and Wilpizeski, C. R. (1966) Neuropharmacological effects of 1,4-butanediol and related congeners compared with those of gamma-hydroxybutyrate and gamma-butyrolactone. *Life Sci.* **5**, 2041–2052.
6. Roth, R. H., Delgado, J. M. R., and Giarman, N. J. (1966) γ-Butyrolactone and γ-hydroxybutyric acid-II. The pharmacologically active form. *Int. J. Neuropharmacol.* **5**, 421–428.
7. Roth, R. H. and Giarman, N. J. (1965) Preliminary report on the metabolism of γ-butyrolactone and γ-hydroxybutyric acid. *Biochem. Pharmacol.* **14**, 177–178.
8. Bustos, G. and Roth, R. H. (1972) Release of monoamines from the striatum and hypothalamus: effect of γ-hydroxybutyrate. *Br. J. Pharmacol.* **46**, 101–115.
9. Roth, R. H. (1975) Gamma-hydroxybutyrate and control of dopaminergic neurons. *Psychopharmacol. Bull.* **11**, 57–58.
10. Murrin, L. C. and Roth, R. H. (1976) Dopaminergic neurons: reversal of effects elicited by γ-butyrolactone by stimulation of the nigro-neostriatal pathway. *Naunyn Schmiedebergs Arch. Pharmacol.* **295**, 15–20.
11. Roth, R. H. (1976) Striatal dopamine and gamma-hydroxybutyrate. *Pharmacol. Ther. B* **2**, 71–88.
12. Sethy, V. H., Roth, R. H., Walters, J. R., Marini, J., and VanWoert, M. H. (1976) Effect of anesthetic doses of γ-hydroxybutyrate on the acetylcholine content of rat brain. *Naunyn Schmiedebergs Arch. Pharmacol.* **295**, 9–14.
13. Madden, T. E. and Johnson, S. W. (1998) Gamma-hydroxybutyrate is a $GABA_B$ receptor agonist that increases a potassium conductance in rat ventral tegmental dopamine neurons. *J. Pharmacol. Exp. Ther.* **287**, 261–265.
14. Roth, R. H., Doherty, J. D., and Walters, J. R. (1980) Gamma-hydroxybutyrate: a role in the regulation of central dopaminergic neurons? *Brain Res.* **189**, 556–560.
15. Diana, M., Mereu, G., Mura, A., Fadda, F., Passino, N., and Gessa, G. (1991) Low doses of γ-hydroxybutyric acid stimulate the firing rate of dopaminergic neurons in unanesthetized rats. *Brain Res.* **566**, 208–211.
15a. Snead, O. C. III. (2000) Evidence for a G protein-coupled gamma-hydroxybutyric acid receptor. *J. Neurochem.* **75**, 1986–1996.
16. Snead, O. C. and Liu, C. C. (1984) Gamma-hydroxybutyric acid binding sites in rat and human brain synaptosomal membranes. *Biochem. Pharmacol.* **33**, 2587–2590.
17. Maitre, M., Hechler, V., Vayer, P., Gobaille, S., Cash, C. D., Schmitt, M., and Bourguignon, J. J. (1990) A specific γ-hydroxybutyrate receptor ligand possesses both antagonistic and anticonvulsant properties. *J. Pharmacol. Exp. Ther.* **255**, 657–663.
18. Snead, O. C. III (1996) Relation of the [^{3}H]γ-hydroxybutyric acid (GHB) binding site to the γ-aminobutyric $acid_B$ ($GABA_B$) receptor in rat brain. *Biochem. Pharmacol.* **52**, 1235–1243.
19. Cash, C. D., Gobaille, S., Kemmel, V., Andriamampandry, C., and Maitre, M. (1999) γ-Hydroxybutyrate receptor function studied by the modulation of nitric oxide synthase activity in rat frontal cortex punches. *Biochem. Pharmacol.* **58**, 1815–1819.
20. Lingenhoehl, K., Brom, R., Heid, J., Beck, P., Froestl, W., Kaupmann, K., et al. (1999) γ-Hydroxybutyrate is a weak agonist at recombinant $GABA_B$ receptors. *Neuropharmacology* **38**, 1667–1673.

21. Takahara, J., Yunoki, S., Yakushiji, W., Yamauchi, J., Yamane, Y., and Ofuji, T. (1977) Stimulatory effects of gamma-hydroxybutyric acid on growth hormone and prolactin release in humans. *J. Clin. Endocrinol. Metab.* **44,** 1014–1017.
22. Van Cauter, E., Plat, L., Scharf, M. B., Leproult, R., Cespedes, S., L'Hermite-Baleriaux, M., and Copinschi, G. (1997) Simultaneous stimulation of slow-wave sleep and growth hormone secretion by gamma-hydroxybutyrate in normal young men. *J. Clin. Invest.* **100,** 745–753.
23. Addolorato, G., Capristo, E., Gessa, G. L., Caputo, F., Stefanini, G. F., and Gasbarrini, G. (1999) Long-term administration of GHB does not affect muscular mass in alcoholics. *Life Sci.* **65,** 191–196.
23a. Vescovi, P. P. and Coiro, V. (2001) Different control of GH secretion by gamma-amino- and gamma-hydroxy-butyric acid in 4-year abstinent alcoholics. *Drug Alcohol Depend.* **61,** 217–221.
23b. Volpi, R., Chiodera, P., Caffarra, P., Scaglioni, A., Malvezzi, L., Saginario, A., and Coiro, V. (2000) Muscarinic cholinergic mediation of the GH response to gamma-hydroxybutyric acid: neuroendocrine evidence in normal and parkinsonian subjects. *Psychoneuroendocrinology* **25,** 179–185.
23c. Rigamonti, A. E. and Müller, E. E. (2000) Gamma-hydroxybutyric acid and growth hormone secretion studies in rats and dogs. *Alcohol* **20,** 293–304.
24. Centers for Disease Control (1990) Multistate outbreak of poisonings associated with illicit use of gamma hydroxybutyrate. *MMWR* **38,** 861–863.
25. Entholzner, E., Mielke, L., Pichlmeier, R., Weber, F., and Schneck, H. (1995) EEG changes during sedation with gamma-hydroxybutyric acid. *Anaesthesist* **44,** 345–350.
26. Lund, L. O., Humphries, J. H., and Virtue, R. W. (1965) Sodium gamma hydroxybutyrate: laboratory and clinical studies. *Can. Anaesth. Soc. J.* **12,** 379–385.
27. Louagie, H. K., Verstraete, A. G., DeSoete, C. J., Baetens, D. G., and Calle, P. A. (1997) A sudden awakening from a near coma after combined intake of gamma-hydroxybutyric acid (GHB) and ethanol. *Clin. Toxicol.* **35,** 591–594.
28. Li, J., Stokes, S. A., and Woeckener, A. (1998) A tale of novel intoxication: seven cases of γ-hydroxybutyric acid overdose. *Ann. Emerg. Med.* **31,** 723–728.
29. Centers for Disease Control and Prevention (1999) Adverse events associated with ingestion of gamma-butyrolactone—Minnesota, New Mexico and Texas, 1998–1999. *MMWR* **48,** 137–140.
30. Marinetti, L. J. and Commissaris, R. L. (1999) The effects of gammahydroxybutyrate (GHB) administration alone and in combination with ethanol on general CNS arousal in rats as measured using the acoustic startle paradigm. Abstract no. 71, Society of Forensic Toxicologists Annual Meeting, San Juan, PR.
31. Marinetti, L. J., Isenschmid, D. S., Hepler, B. R., Schmidt, C. J., Somerset, J. S., and Kanluen, S. (2000) Two gamma-hydroxybutyric acid (GHB) fatalities. Abstract K16, American Academy of Forensic Science Annual Meeting, Reno, NV.
32. Ferrara, S. D., Tedeschi, L., Frison, G., and Rossi, A. (1995) Fatality due to gamma-hydroxybutyric acid (GHB) and heroin intoxication. *JFSCA* **40,** 501–504.
33. ElSohly, M. A. and Salamone, S. J. (1999) Prevalence of drugs used in cases of alleged sexual assault. *J. Analyt. Toxicol.* **23,** 141–146.

34. Hernandez, M., McDaniel, C. H., Costanza, C. D., and Hernandez, O. J. (1998) GHB-induced delirium: a case report and review of the literature on gamma hydroxybutyric acid. *Am. J. Drug Alcohol Abuse* **24,** 179–183.
35. Craig, K., Gomez, H. F., McManus, J. L., and Bania, T. C. (2000) Severe gamma-hydroxybutyrate withdrawal: a case report and literature review. *J. Emerg. Med.* **18,** 65–70.
36. Dyer, J. E., Roth, B., and Hyma, B. A. (2001) Gamma-hydroxybutyrate withdrawal syndrome. *Ann. Emerg. Med.* **37,** 147–153.
37. Kleinschmidt, S., Schellhase, C., and Mertzlufft, F. (1999) Continuous sedation during spinal anaesthesia: gamma-hydroxybutyrate vs. propofol. *Eur. J. Anaesthesiol.* **16,** 23–30.
38. *Pharmacy Today* (2000) 'Acquaintance rape drug' may one day help instead of hurt, pp. 17.
39. Lammers, G. J., Van Dijk, J. G., Ferrari, M. D., Van Gerven, J. M., Declerck, A. C., and Trost, J. (1999) Gammahydroxybutyrate must remain available for patients with narcolepsy. *Ned Tijdschr Geneeskd* **143,** 2062–2063.
39a. Feldman, N. T. (2000) Gamma-hydroxybutyric acid in the right hands. *South. Med. J.* **93,** 1037–1038.
40. Broughton, R. and Mamelak, M. (1979) The treatment of narcolepsy-cataplexy with nocturnal gamma-hydroxybutyrate. *J. Can. Des Sci. Neurol.* **6,** 1–6.
40a. Colombo, G., Agabio, R., Lobina, C., Reali, R., Fadda, F., and Gessa, G. L. (1995) Cross-tolerance to ethanol and γ-hydroxybutyric acid. *Eur. J. Pharmacol.* **273,** 235–238.
41. Addolorato, G., Castelli, E., Stefanini, G. F., Casella, G., Caputo, F., Marsigli, L., Bernardi, M., Gasbarrini, G., and GHB Study Group (1996) An open multicentric study evaluating 4-hydroxybutyric acid sodium salt in the medium-term treatment of 179 alcohol dependent subjects. *Alcohol Alcoholism* **31,** 341–345.
42. Agabio, R., Colombo, G., Loche, A., Lobina, C., Pani, M. L., Reali, R., and Gessa, G. L. (1998) γ-Hydroxybutyric acid reducing effect on ethanol intake: evidence in favour of a substitution mechanism. *Alcohol Alcoholism* **33,** 465–474.
43. Poldrugo, F. and Addolorato, G. (1999) The role of gamma-hydroxybutyric acid in the treatment of alcoholism: from animal to clinical studies. *Alcohol Alcoholism* **34,** 15–24.
44. Colombo, G., Agabio, R., Lobina, C., Loche, A., Reali, R., and Gessa, G. L. (1998) High sensitivity to γ-hydroxybutyric acid in ethanol-preferring sP rats. *Alcohol Alcoholism* **33,** 121–125.
45. Addolorato, G., Caputo, F., Stefanini, G. F., and Gasbarrini, G. (1997b) Gamma-hydroxybutyric acid in the treatment of alcohol dependence: possible craving development for the drug. *Addiction* **92,** 1041–1042.
45a. Beghè, F. and Carpanini, M. T. (2000) Safety and tolerability of gamma-hydroxybutyric acid in the treatment of alcohol-dependent patients. *Alcohol* **20,** 223–225.
46. Gallimberti, L., Cibin, M., Pagin, P., Sabbion, R., Pani, P. P., Pirastu, R., et al. (1993) Gamma-hydroxybutyric acid for treatment of opiate withdrawal syndrome. *Neuropsychopharmacology* **9,** 77–81.

GHB and Its Analogs

46a. Fattore, L., Martellotta, M. C., Cossu, G., and Fratta, W. (2000) Gamma-hydroxybutyric acid an evaluation of its rewarding properties in rats and mice. *Alcohol* **20**, 247–256.
47. Scharf, M. B., Hauck, M., Stover, R., McDannold, M., and Berkowitz, D. (1998) Effect of gamma-hydroxybutyrate on pain, fatigue and the alpha sleep anomaly in patients with fibromyalgia: preliminary report. *J. Rheumatol.* **25**, 1986–1990.
48. 106th Congress (2000) Hillory J. Farias and Samantha Reid Date-Rape Drug Prohibiton Act of 2000. Public Law 106–172.
48a. Federal Registery (2000) Placement of gamma-butyrolactone in List I of the Controlled Substances Act (21 U.S.C. 802(34)). Drug Enforcement Administration, Justice. Final Rule. Apr. 24; 65(79), 21,645–21,647.
48b. DEA Southwest Laboratory in San Diego, California (2001) Solid GBL in Southern California. *Microgram* **34**, 45.
49. Food and Drug Administration (1999) FDA warns about products containing gamma butyrolactone or GBL and asks companies to issue a recall. *FDA Talk Paper*, January 21, T99-5.
49a. γ-Butyrolactone (1999) *IARC Monogr. Eval. Carcinog. Risks Human (1987)* **71** (Pt.2) 367–382.
49b. Morris, J. A. (2000) Potential for gamma-butyrolactone synthesis from tetrahydrofuran and 1,4-butanediol. *Microgram* **33**, 321–324.
50. Arena, C. and Fung, H. L. (1980) Absorption of sodium γ-hydroxybutyrate and its prodrug γ-butyrolactone: relationship between in vitro transport and in vivo absorption. *J. Pharmaceut. Sci.* **69**, 356–358.
51. Lettieri, J. and Fung, H. L. (1978) Improved pharmacological activity via prodrug modification comparitive pharmacokinetics of sodium gamma-hydroxybutyrate and gamma-butyrolactone. *Res. Commun. Chem. Pathol. Pharmacol.* **22**, 107–118.
51a. Gianutsos, G. and Moore, K. E. (1978) Tolerance to the effects of baclofen and γ-butyrolactone on locomotor activity and dopaminergic neurons in the mouse. *J. Pharmacol. Exper. Therap.* **207**, 859–869.
51b. Gianutsos, G. and Suzdak, P. D. (1984) Evidence for down-regulation of GABA receptors following long-term gamma-butyrolactone. *Naunyn-Schmiedebergs Arch. Pharmacol.* **328**, 62–68.
51c. Kraner, J. C., Plassard, J. W., McCoy, D. J., Rorabeck, J. A., Witeck, M. J., Smith, K. B., and Evans, M. A. (2000) A death from ingestion of 1,4-butanediol, a GHB precursor. Poster 39, Program and Abstracts of the Society of Forensic Toxicologists annual meeting, Milwaukee, WI.
51d. Zvosec, D. L., Smith, S. W., McCutcheon, J. R., Spillane, J., Hall, B. J., and Peacock, E. A. (2001) Adverse events, including death, associated with the use of 1,4-butanediol. *N. Engl. J. Med.* **344**, 87–93.
52. Dyer, J. E. (2000) Personal communication.
53. FDA talk paper (1999) FDA warns about GBL-related products, May 11, T99-21.
54. Kaufman, E. E., Relkin, N., and Nelson, T. (1983) Regulation and properties of an $NADP^+$ oxidoreductase which functions as a γ-hydroxybutyrate dehydrogenase. *J. Neurochem.* **40**, 1639–1646.

55. Kaufman, E. E. and Nelson, T. (1987) Evidence for the participation of a cytosolic NADP+-dependent oxidoreductase in the catabolism of γ-hydroxybutyrate in vivo. *J. Neurochem.* **48,** 1935–1941.
56. Kaufman, E. E., Nelson, T., Goochee, C., and Sokoloff, L. (1979) Purification and characterization of an NADP+-linked alcohol oxido-reductase which catalyzes the interconversion of γ-hydroxybutyrate and succinic semialdehyde. *J. Neurochem.* **32,** 699–712.
57. Bessman, S. P. and McCabe R. B. III. (1972) 1,4-butanediol—a substrate for rat liver and horse liver alcohol dehydrogenases. *Biochem. Pharmacol.* **21,** 1135–1142.
58. Doherty, J. D., Stout, R. W., and Roth, R. H. (1975) Metabolism of [1-^{14}C] γ-hydroxybutyric acid by rat brain after intraventricular injection. *Biochem. Pharmacol.* **24,** 469–474.
59. Baselt, R. C. (2000) *Disposition of Toxic Drugs and Chemicals in Man,* 5th edit., Chemical Toxicology Institute, Foster City, CA, pp. 386–388.
60. Kaufman, E. E. and Nelson, T. (1991) An overview of γ-hydroxybutyrate catabolism: the role of the cytosolic NADP+-dependent oxidoreductase EC 1.1.1.19 and of a mitochondrial hydroxyacid-oxoacid transhydrogenase in the initial, rate-limiting step in this pathway. *Neurochem. Res.* **16,** 965–974.
61. Gibson, K. M., Hoffman, G. F., Hodson, A. K., Bottiglieri, T., and Jakobs, C. (1998) 4-Hydroxybutyric acid and the clinical phenotype of succinic semialdehyde dehydrogenase deficiency: an inborn error of GABA metabolism. *Neuropediatrics* **29,** 14–22.
62. Roth, R. H. and Giarman, N. J. (1966) γ-Butyrolactone and γ-hydroxybutyric acid—I. Distribution and metabolism. *Biochem. Pharmacol.* **15,** 1333–1348.
63. Irwin, R. D. (1996) *NTP Summary Report on the Metabolism, Disposition, and Toxicity of 1,4-Butanediol.* NIH Publication No. 96-3932, May, Toxicology Report Series Number 54.
64. Snead, O. C. III, Brown, G. B., and Morawetz, R. B. (1981) Concentration of gamma-hydroxybutyric acid in ventricular and lumbar cerebrospinal fluid. *N. Engl. J. Med.* **304,** 93–95.
65. Nelson, T., Kaufman, E., Kline, J., and Sokoloff, L. (1981) The extraneural distribution of γ-hydroxybutyrate. *J. Neurochem.* **37,** 1345–1348.
66. Doherty, J. D., Hattox, S. E., Snead, O. C., and Roth, R. H. (1978) Identification of endogenous γ-hydroxybutyrate in human and bovine brain and its regional distribution in human, guinea pig and Rhesus monkey brain. *J. Pharmacol. Exp. Ther.* **207,** 130–139.
67. Shumate, J. S. and Snead, O. C. III. (1979) Plasma and central nervous system kinetics of gamma-hydroxybutyrate. *Res. Commun. Chem. Path. Pharmacol.* **25,** 241–256.
67a. Snead, O. C. III, Yu, R. K., and Huttenlocher, P. R. (1976) Gamma hydroxybutyrate correlation of serum and cerebrospinal fluid levels with electroencephalographic and behavioral effects. *Neurology* **26,** 51–56.
68. Ferrara, S. D., Tedeschi, L., Frison, G., Castagna, F., Gallimberti, L., Giorgetti, R., et al. (1993) Therapeutic gamma-hydroxybutyric acid monitoring in plasma and

urine by gas chromatography-mass spectrometry. *J. Pharmaceut. Biomed. Anal.* **11,** 483–487.
69. Van der Pol, W., Van der Kleijn, E., and Lauw, M. (1975) Gas chromatographic determination and pharmacokinetics of 4-hydroxybutyrate in dog and mouse. *J. Pharmacokin. Biopharmaceut.* **3,** 99–113.
70. Ferrara, S. D., Zotti, S., Tedeschi, L., Frison, G., Castagna, F., Gallimberti, L., et al. (1992) Pharmacokinetics of γ-hydroxybutyric acid in alcohol dependent patients after single and repeated oral doses. *Br. J. Clin. Pharmacol.* **34,** 231–235.
70a. Borgen, L. A., Lai, A., and Okerholm, R. A. (2001) Xyrem® (sodium oxybate): the effects of gender and food on plasma kinetics. Orphan Medical, Inc., Minnetonka, MN, personal communication.
71. Lettieri, J. and Fung, H. L. (1978) Improved pharmacological activity via prodrug modification; comparative pharmacokinetics of sodium gamma-hydroxybutyrate and gamma-butyrolactone. *Res. Commun. Chem. Pathol. Pharmacol.* **22,** 107–118.
72. Eli, M. and Cattabeni, F. (1983) Endogenous gamma-hydroxybutyrate in rat brain areas: postmortem changes and effects of drugs interfering with gamma-aminobutyric acid metabolism. *J. Neurochem.* **41,** 524–530.
73. *The Merck Index* (1996) 12th edit., Merck & Co., Whitehouse Station, NJ, pp. 1366–1367.
74. Seiler, N. (1980) On the role of GABA in vertebrate polyamine metabolism. *Physiol. Chem. Phys.* **12,** 411–429.
74a. Sessa, A. and Perin, A. (1994) Diamine oxidase in relation to diamine and polyamine metabolism. *Agents Actions* **43,** 69–77.
75. Snead, O. C. III, Liu, C., and Bearden, L. J. (1982) Studies on the relation of γ-hydroxybutyric acid (GHB) to γ-aminobutyric acid (GABA)—evidence that GABA is not the sole source for GHB in rat brain. *Biochem. Pharmacol.* **31,** 3917–3923.
76. Stephens, B. G., Coleman, D. E., and Baselt, R. C. (1999) In vitro stability of endogenous gamma-hydroxybutyrate in postmortem blood. *J. Forensic Sci.* **44,** 231.
77. Anderson, D. T. and Kuwahara, T. (1997) Endogenous gamma hydroxybutyrate (GHB) levels in postmortem specimens. Presented at the combined meeting of CAT/NWAFS/SWAFS/SAT in Las Vegas, NV, November 7.
78. Fieler, E. L., Coleman, D. E., and Baselt, R. C. (1998) γ-Hydroxybutyrate concentrations in pre- and postmortem blood and urine. *Clin. Chem.* **44,** 692.
78a. LeBeau, M. A., Montgomery, M. A., Jufer, R. A., and Miller, M. L. (2000) Elevated GHB in citrate-buffered blood. *J. Analyt. Toxicol.* **24,** 383–384.
79. Ciolino, L. A. and Mesmer, M. Z. (2000) Bridging the gap between GHB and GBL —forensic issues of interconversion. Abstr. B51, American Academy of Forensic Science Annual Meeting, Reno, NV.
79a. Anderson, D. T., Muto, J. J., and Andrews, J. M. (2000) Case report: postmortem tissue distribution of gamma hydroxybutyrate (GHB) and gamma butyrolactone (GBL) in a single fatality. Poster 37, Program and Abstracts of the Society of Forensic Toxicologists annual meeting, Milwaukee, WI.
80. McCutcheon, J. R., Hall, B. J., Schroeder, P. M., Peacock, E. A., and Bayardo, R. J. (2000) Fatal intoxication following recreational ingestion of 1,4-butanediol. Abstr. K15, American Academy of Forensic Science Annual Meeting, Reno, NV.

81. LeBeau, M. A., Montgomery, M. A., Miller, M. L., and Burmeister, S. G. (1999) Analysis of biofluids for gamma-hydroxybutyrate (GHB) and gamma-butyrolactone (GBL) by headspace GC/FID and GC/MS. Presented in part at the 26th Annual Meeting, Society of Forensic Toxicologists, Rio Mar, Puerto Rico.
82. Anderson, D. A. (1997) Gamma hydroxybutyrate (GHB) analysis, Los Angeles County Coroner's Department, Toxicology Laboratory, personal communication.
83. Couper, F. J. and Logan, B. K. (2000) Determination of γ-hydroxybutyrate (GHB) in biological specimens by gas chromatography-mass spectrometry. *J. Analyt. Toxicol.* **24,** 1–7.
84. Elian, A. A. (2000) A novel method for GHB detection in urine and its application in drug-facilitated sexual assaults. *Forensic Sci. Int.* **109,** 183–187.
85. Andollo, W. and Hearn, W. L. (1998) The characterization of drugs used in sexual battery—the Dade County experience. Abstract K52, American Academy of Forensic Sciences annual meeting, San Francisco, California.
86. McCusker, R. R., Paget-Wilkes, H., Chronister, C. W., Goldberger, B. A., and ElSohly, M. A. (1999) Analysis of gamma-hydroxybutyrate (GHB) in urine by gas chromatography-mass spectrometry, *J. Analyt. Toxicol.* **23,** 301–305.
87. Crifasi, J. A. and Telepchak, M. (2000) A solid phase method for gamma-hydroxybutyrate (GHB) in blood, urine, vitreous or tissue without conversion to gamma-butyrolactone (GBL) using United Chemical Technologies' ZSGHB020 or CSGHB203 solid phase extraction columns—personal communication.
88. Biochemical Diagnostics (2000) Method for the measurement of gamma-hydroxybutyrate (GHB) in blood and urine using GC/MS—personal communication.
89. Ehrhardt, J. D., Vayer, P. H., and Maitre, M. (1988) A rapid and sensitive method for the determination of γ-hydroxybutyric acid and trans-γ-hydroxycrotonic acid in rat brain tissue by gas chromatography/mass spectrometry with negative ion detection. *Biomed. Environm. Mass Spectrom.* **15,** 521–524.
90. Frison, G., Tedeschi, L, Maietti, S., and Ferrara, S. D. (1998) Determination of gamma-hydroxy-butyric acid (GHB) in plasma and urine by headspace solid-phase microextraction (SPME) and gas chromatography-positive ion chemical ionization-mass spectrometry. Proceedings of the 1998 Joint Society of Forensic Toxicologists and The International Association of Forensic Toxicologists SOFT/TIAFT International Meeting (Spiehler, V., ed.), pp. 394–404.
91. Barker, S. A., Snead, O. C., Poldrugo, F., Liu, C., Fish, F. P., and Settine, R. L. (1985) Identification and quantitation of 1,4-butanediol in mammalian tissues: an alternative biosynthetic pathway for gamma-hydroxybutyric acid. *Biochem. Pharmacol.* **34,** 1849–1852.

Chapter 7

Analysis of Urine Samples in Cases of Alleged Sexual Assault
Case History

*Mahmoud A. ElSohly, Luen F. Lee,
Lynn B. Holzhauer, and Salvatore J. Salamone*

1. INTRODUCTION

The development of sensitive and specific analytical techniques and procedures has always been a cornerstone in forensic toxicology to establish scientific facts relevant to specific cases. The importance of such sensitive and credible procedures has gained a new dimension over the last few years in countering media inaccuracies and exaggerations concerning certain forensic issues, most recently exemplified by reports on the use of drugs in cases of alleged sexual assault.

The media has made great play of the concept of "date rape" or "acquaintance rape," that is, the use of drugs by friends or acquaintances of the victim to facilitate sexual assault *(1,2)*. A number of drugs have been implicated by the media in such alleged criminal activities, among them γ-hydroxybutyrate (GHB) *(3,4)*, ketamine *(5)*, and flunitrazepam *(6,7)*.

Flunitrazepam, a member of the benzodiazepine class of compounds, has been marketed for more than 20 yr and is a safe and efficacious drug for the treatment of severe and debilitating sleep disorders. It is among the most frequently prescribed hypnotics in many countries, but it has never been available in the United States, for purely commercial reasons.

From: *Forensic Science: Benzodiazepines and GHB: Detection and Pharmacology*
Edited by: S. J. Salamone © Humana Press Inc., Totowa, NJ

It has, however, been smuggled into the United States, although reported instances of unlawful imports, distribution, and abuse have been largely limited to two states, Florida and Texas. There seems to have been a decrease in illegal trafficking in the last few years, so that flunitrazepam abuse appears to have been a short-lived "fashion" among the young and polydrug users.

Stories of the misuse of flunitrazepam to commit sexual assaults began to appear in the United States media in the mid-1990s, but the number of cases in which it was implicated was very small. Reports of sexual assaults using drugs emerged in other countries, too—and continue to do so from time to time—but it is often impossible to sort out fact from fantasy and inaccurate, sensationalized reporting.

The major manufacturer of flunitrazepam, under the brand name Rohypnol, is F. Hoffmann-La Roche (Roche), although there are several other manufacturers. Despite the fact that very few reported cases of assault associated with flunitrazepam have been substantiated, Roche took a number of steps to minimize the potential for abuse of its product and actively collaborated with international drug regulatory and law enforcement agencies. Among those measures was a reduction in dose and package size and the introduction of a reformulated, color-releasing tablet.

Roche also sought to determine the facts about the use of drugs, including flunitrazepam, in alleged cases of sexual assault, notably by sponsoring the development of sensitive analytical techniques to enable flunitrazepam to be detected in urine samples. Subsequently, a testing program was set up to offer wholly independent urine analyses to victims of alleged sexual assault in the United States.

The method developed for the purpose of detecting flunitrazepam in urine samples submitted under the Roche program was a very specific and sensitive gas chromatography/mass spectrometry (GC/MS) procedure *(8)*. The procedure was sensitive to less than 1 ng/mL of the major urinary metabolite of flunitrazepam (7-amino-flunitrazepam). This sensitivity allowed the detection of the drug in urine for at least 72 h post-ingestion of as low a dose as 1 mg of flunitrazepam.

This case history outlines the analytical techniques involved and the results of more than 3000 urinalyses during the 4-yr testing program.

2. RECEIPT OF SPECIMENS FOR ANALYSIS

ElSohly Laboratories, Incorporated (ELI) of Oxford, Mississippi, was selected by Roche to analyze all samples collected from alleged sexual assault victims under its public service offering. Information on the availability of the service was distributed by Roche to rape crisis centers, law enforcement agencies, and emergency rooms throughout the United States. These agencies were advised that urine specimens should be collected and handled under standard forensic chain of custody procedures and that the contract laboratory would analyze each specimen for alcohol, flunitrazepam, and other benzodiazepines, amphetamines, barbiturates, cocaine, GHB, marijuana, and opiates. Other drugs of abuse were tested such as propoxyphene, methaqualone, and phencyclidine (PCP). While Roche paid for all testing and literature distributed to the submitting agencies, it emphasized that it had no influence whatsoever on the specimen collection or the testing results. Roche's sole interest in the program to was ascertain scientific facts relative to the prevalence of drugs of abuse in these alleged sexual assault cases. Further, the agencies were advised that doses of a single 1-mg tablet of flunitrazepam were detectable in the urine for up to 72 h post-ingestion. On receipt at the testing laboratory, the specimens were refrigerated prior to testing and were stored at −20°C after testing.

3. TESTING PROTOCOL

The testing protocol involved the following distinct steps:

1. All specimens were screened by OnLine immunoassay (Roche Diagnostic Corporation, Indianapolis, IN) for nine different drug classes. The immunoassays were performed at the manufacturer's recommended cutoff levels for amphetamines at 1000 ng/mL, barbiturates at 200 ng/mL, cocaine metabolite at 300 ng/mL, cannabinoids at 50 ng/mL, methaqualone at 300 ng/mL, opiates at 300 ng/mL, phencyclidine at 25 ng/mL, and propoxyphene at 300 ng/mL. The benzodiazepine assay was performed following a previously published procedure using a 50 ng/mL cutoff and β-glucuronidase pretreatment *(9)*.
2. Specimens were screened for benzodiazepines by a second immunoassay (either OnTrak or TestStik, both manufactured by Roche Diagnostic Corporation). These assays have a different cross-reactivity profile than the OnLine immunoassay for benzodiazepines. The analysis was performed following the manufacturer's protocol.
3. Any specimen screening positive for any drug class was confirmed by GC/MS analysis following the laboratory's standard operating procedures for the different drugs. GC/MS analysis for the different drug classes was carried out using liquid/liquid extraction procedures in the presence of appropriate internal standards (primarily deuterated analogs of the different analytes). The cannabinoids assay was directed toward 11-nor-Δ^9-THC-9-COOH; the cocaine assay was directed toward benzoylecgonine; the opiates assay toward morphine (total) and codeine; the amphetamines toward amphetamine and methamphetamine; propoxyphene assay toward both propoxyphene and norpropoxyphene; the barbiturate assay toward butalbital, secobarbital, pentobarbital, butabarbital, and phenobarbital; while the assays for PCP

and methaqualone were directed toward the parent drugs. The benzodiazepines GC/MS confirmation method was based on acid hydrolysis of the urine specimen to convert all benzodiazepine metabolites of similar basic skeleton to the same benzophenone. The benzophenones monitored were those derived from norfludiazepam, bromazepam, nitrazepam, diazepam, oxazepam, alprazolam, triazolam, and lorazepam. Therefore, any benzodiazepine giving rise to any of these benzophenones was reported as the basic benzodiazepine producing such benzophenone. For example, a positive finding for the benzophenone corresponding to oxazepam was reported as positive for oxazepam, but the urine could actually contain oxazepam or any related benzodiazepine that would produce the same benzophenone upon acid hydrolysis. Other benzodiazepines that could produce the same benzophenone as oxazepam would include nordiazepam, clorazepate, oxazolam, chlordiazepoxide, and others such as α-OH-alprazolam. Therefore, the interpretation of the GC/MS confirmation results should be done with care, and if it is really necessary to identify the specific benzodiazepine responsible for the positive test, a second GC/MS analysis would be necessary using only enzyme hydrolysis prior to reextraction.

4. All specimens were analyzed by GC/MS for GHB. The analysis was carried out using a minor modification of the procedure previously reported by Ferrara et al. *(10)*. In brief, 2 mL of urine were treated with 0.5 mL of 20% trifluoroacetic acid at 75°C for 1 h, using γ-valerolactone as the internal standard. After cooling to room temperature, the reaction mixture was adjusted to pH 6.5 with 2 N NaOH and then extracted with 3 mL of $CHCl_3$. The chloroform extract was used for GC/MS analysis without further concentration. A DB-5 MS column (25 m × 0.2 mm, 0.33 µm film) was operated at 60°C (1 min) to 90°C at 10°C/min, then up to 275°C at 35°C/min with a temperature hold of 1 min before reequilibration. The ions monitored were at m/z 42, 56, and 86 for GHB and 56, 41, and 85 for the internal standard. A calibration curve from 10 to 50 µg/mL was used for quantitation using the peak area ratio of ions 42 (drug) and 56 (internal standard). This analytical procedure converts GHB to γ-buterolactone (GBL) prior to extraction.

5. All specimens were analyzed by GC/FID for ethanol. The analysis was carried out using direct injection of a 1-µL volume of a mixture of 100 µL of the urine specimen and 100 µL of internal standard (IS) solution (100 mg/dL of isopropanol) into a GC equipped with a 6 ft × 2 mm ID 60/80 carbopack/5% and operated at 80°C. The quantitation was performed by comparing the area ratio of ethanol/IS relative to a calibration curve from 20–120 mg/dL of ethanol.

6. All specimens were analyzed by GC/MS for flunitrazepam metabolites, regardless of the results of the benzodiazepines screen. The analysis was carried out following the procedure previously reported by ElSohly et al. *(8)*. This procedure used an acid hydrolysis step which converts flunitrazepam and metabolites to their corresponding benzophenones. The limit of detection was less than 1 ng/mL of 7-amino-flunitrazepam which was found to be the major urinary metabolite *(8,9)*. Initially, the internal standard was d_5-oxazepam which was subsequently changed to d_3-7-amino-flunitrazepam when the latter became commercially available.

Urine Sample Analysis

The use of this GC/MS procedure to analyze each and every urine specimen submitted under this program (more than 3000), coupled with the fact that more than 98% of the samples were collected within 72 h of the alleged incident, assured that flunitrazepam would be detected had it been used at the time of the incident.

4. RESULTS AND DISCUSSION

A total of 3303 urine specimens were submitted to ElSohly Laboratories for testing under this program. The main objective was to provide independent analyses to determine the facts relative to the use of drugs, including flunitrazepam, in these cases of alleged sexual assault. Therefore, specimens had to meet two criteria to be tested under the program: there had to be an allegation that a drug had been administered to the claimant prior to the alleged sexual assault, and the specimen had to have been collected within 72 h of the alleged incident.

The 72-h window was selected to ensure that if flunitrazepam had been administered, its metabolite(s) would be detected, given the sensitivity of the GC/MS method used *(8)*.

Figure 1 shows the distribution of the specimens analyzed under this program within different time intervals from alleged drug ingestion to specimen collection. Among the 3303 specimens analyzed, there were 3262 specimens collected within 72 h of the incident (98.8%), and 2411 specimens (73%) were collected within 24 h. Figure 2 shows the number of positive samples confirmed by GC/MS for the different drug classes. None of the drugs tested for was detected in 1277 samples (38.7%), and the remaining 61.3% of the samples were positive for one or more drugs. Of all 2026 positives, there were 1358 samples positive for alcohol (67% of all positives or 41.1% of all specimens tested), making alcohol the most predominant substance found in the submitted specimens.

The second most predominant drug was marijuana with 613 samples positive (30.3% of all positives or 18.6% of all specimens tested). Benzodiazepines as a general class were identified in 313 cases (9.5% of all specimens collected) of which 11 specimens were positive for flunitrazepam. Cocaine was found in 279 samples (8.4%) and amphetamines in 220 samples (6.7%). GHB was found in 100 samples (3.03%), opiates in 87 samples (2.63%), propoxyphene in 44 samples (1.33%), barbiturates in 40 samples (1.21%), and PCP in 3 samples only (<0.1%). No samples tested positive for methaqualone.

The distribution of the positive benzodiazepine samples among the different subclasses is shown in Fig. 3. As could be expected, the majority of the

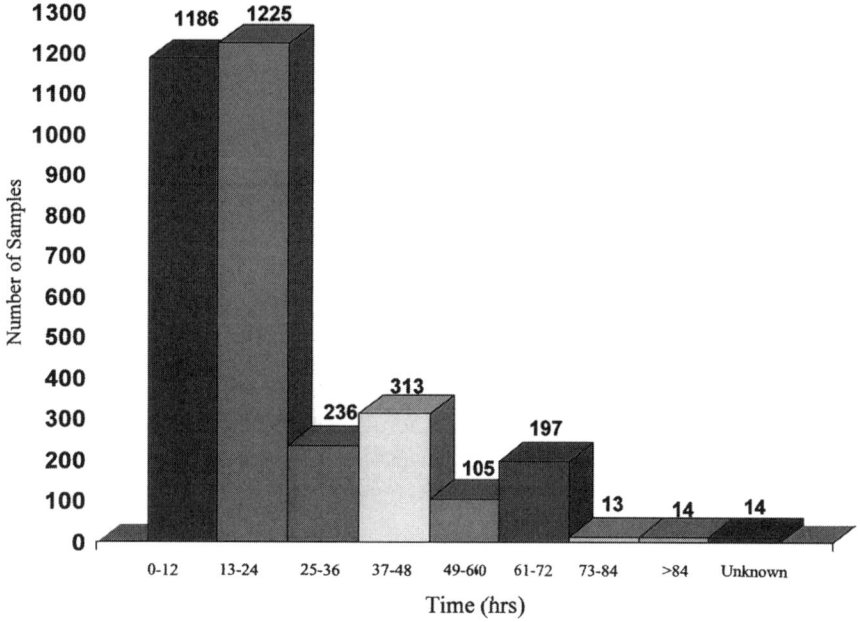

Note: If time interval is a span, the midpoint is used.

Fig. 1. Time interval from alleged drug ingestion to collection of samples.

samples (71.7%) were confirmed by GC/MS for the oxazepam and diazepam subclasses since these have the most common basic skeleton to many benzodiazepines. There were only two samples positive for benzodiazepines which could not be classified among the subclasses tested, and therefore these were labeled unspecified (benzo unspec) in Fig. 3. The next most common benzodiazepine among positives was clonazepam, identified as 7-amino-clonazepam in >10% of all benzodiazepine positives. On the other hand, flunitrazepam, which was alleged to be the "date-rape drug," was found in only 11 specimens (0.33% of all specimens tested). Even then, flunitrazepam was found along with other drugs in six specimens and only found alone in five specimens. Table 1 shows the specifics of the 11 cases in which flunitrazepam was detected. Several observations can be made from Table 1: *(1)* Not all the specimens screened positive for benzodiazepines, even with the sensitive (50 ng/mL cutoff) OnLine immunoassay. Therefore, unless a sensitive method such as GC/MS or a more specific immunoassay is used to screen urine samples, flunitrazepam positives could go undetected; *(2)* several samples were positive for at least one other drug and as many as five other drugs; *(3)* the five samples containing flunitraz-

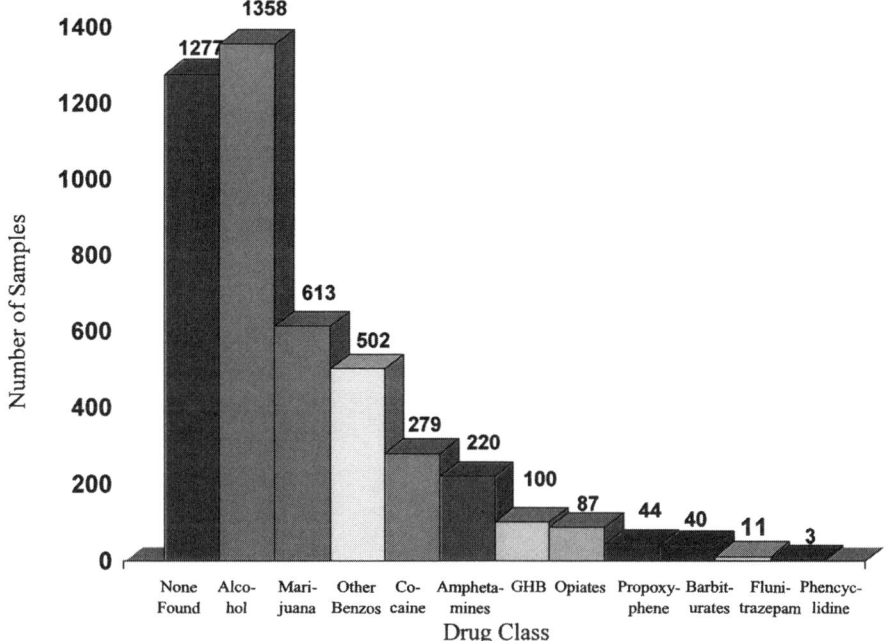

Fig. 2. Distribution of positives confirmed by GC/MS in 3303 samples for different drug classes. Some samples contain more than one substance.

epam alone were collected 12–25 h after the incident. Because of the time lag with these five specimens, the involvement of alcohol in these cases cannot be discounted, considering its rapid clearance from the body. It must be emphasized that the fact that a very sensitive GC/MS procedure with an LoD of <1 ng/mL was used for the analysis of all specimens for flunitrazepam metabolites means that it can be confidently stated that no flunitrazepam positive went undetected.

Examination of the results of this study further shows that a high percentage of the samples tested positive for more than one drug, indicating multiple drug use. Table 2 shows the frequency of occurrence of multiple positives among individual samples, and Table 3 shows the distribution of samples with multiple drug use.

Among the three most predominant drugs (alcohol, marijuana, and benzodiazepines), the following shows their relationship with respect to other drug use. Of the 1358 alcohol positive samples, 246 were positive for marijuana, 131 were positive for cocaine, 119 were positive for benzodiazepines of which 3 contained flunitrazepam, 45 were positive for GHB, 38 were positive for

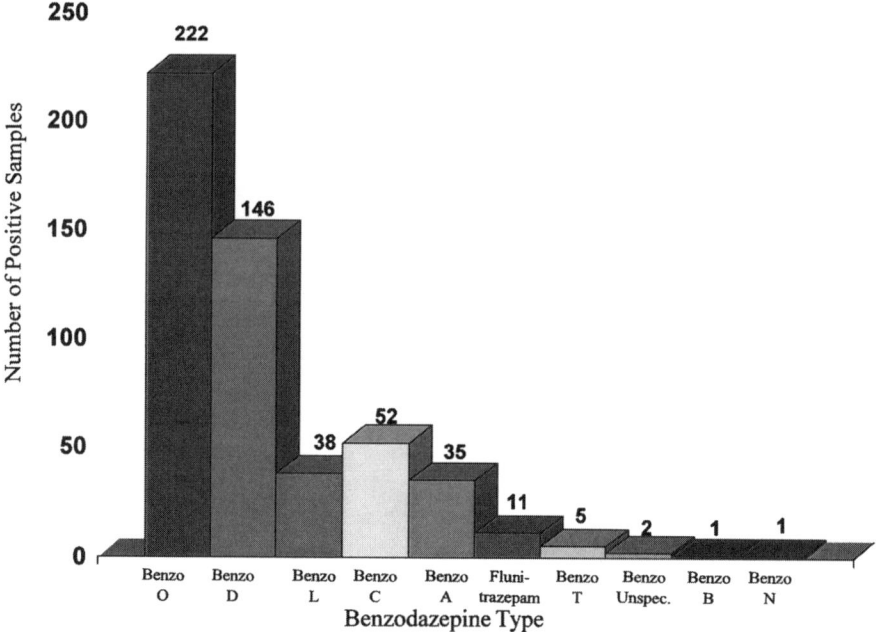

Fig. 3. Distribution of positive benzodiazepines among the different subclasses. Some samples contain more than one substance.

amphetamines, 24 were positive for opiates, 19 were positive for propoxyphene, and 9 were positive for barbiturates. Of the 613 marijuana positive samples, 246 were positive for alcohol, 111 were positive for cocaine, 97 were positive for benzodiazepines of which 2 contained flunitrazepam, 52 were positive for amphetamines, 22 were positive for GHB, 15 were positive for opiates, 11 were positive for propoxyphene, and 7 were positive for barbiturates. Among the 304 samples positive for benzodiazepines, 116 were positive for alcohol, 95 were positive for marijuana, 56 were positive for cocaine, 28 were positive for amphetamines, 22 were positive for opiates, 17 were positive for GHB, 16 were positive for barbiturates, and 15 were positive for propoxyphene.

It must be mentioned that the 304 other benzodiazepine positive samples shown in Table 3 were actually positive for 502 individual benzodiazepine subclasses as shown in Fig. 2, indicating multibenzodiazepine positives within the same samples.

All 50 states provided specimens for the study. Figure 4 shows a map of the United States with the number of samples received from each state. The states with the highest number of samples were California (413 samples), Texas (379 samples), New York (196 samples), Florida (174 samples), Pennsylvania

Table 1
Details of Specimens Identified as Flunitrazepam Positive

Origin	Time post-incident (h)	Benzodiazephines screen	GC/MS 7-amino-flunitrazepam (ng/mL)	GC/MS 7-amino-nor-flunitrazepam (ng/mL)	Other drugs detected
TX	24	Positive	580	75.7	
TX	12	Negative	463	59.8	
OH	24	Positive	403	27.9	Benzoylecgonine @ 32,600 ng/mL; oxazepam @ 36.8 ng/mL; diazepam @ 25.8 ng/mL
FL	13	Positive	787	58.0	THC-COOH @ 153 ng/mL
CA	20	Negative	55.2	8.4	
OK	22	Positive	457	40.8	
TX	12	Positive	349	63.8	Ethanol @ 6.2 mg/dL; THC-COOH @ 48 ng/mL; benzoylecgonine @ 790 ng/mL; bromazepam @ 1020 ng/mL; oxazepam @ 1747 ng/mL
TX	8	Negative	9.9	2.5	Ethanol @ 131 mg/dL
AR	24	Positive	287	306	
MN	18	Positive	71.9	59.7	Benzoylecgonine @ 2339 ng/mL
TX	10–13	Positive	677	744	Ethanol @ 7.5 mg/dL; benzoylecgonine @ 12,680 ng/mL; codeine @ 206 ng/mL; morphine @ 6644 ng/mL

Table 2
Frequency of Multiple Positive Results Among the Samples Analyzed

Number of positive results	Count	Total samples ($n = 3303$)	Total positive samples ($n = 2026$)
None	1277	38.7%	
One	1288	39.0%	63.6%
Two or more	738	22.3%	36.4%
Two	451	13.7%	22.3%
Three	162	4.9%	8.0%
Four	71	2.1%	3.5%
Five	33	1.0%	1.6%
Six	16	0.5%	0.8%
Seven	4	0.1%	0.2%

Table 3
Distribution of Samples
with More Than One Positive Test Result by Primary Drug Class

Samples positive for		Also tested positive for								
	N^a	EtOH	AMPS	BARBS	FN	COC	GHB	THC	OPI	BENZO	PPXY
Alcohol	1358	—	38	9	3	131	45	246	24	116	19
AMP	116	38	—	1	0	15	9	52	6	28	1
BARB	39	9	1	—	0	2	1	7	5	16	2
BENZO/FN	11	3	0	0	—	4	0	2	1	2	0
COC	279	131	15	2	4	—	12	111	20	56	6
GHB	100	45	9	1	0	12	—	22	3	17	0
THC	613	246	52	7	2	111	22	—	15	95	11
OPI	56	24	6	5	1	20	3	15	—	22	4
Other BENZO	304	116	28	16	2	56	17	95	22	—	15
PPXY	44	19	1	2	0	6	0	11	4	15	—

^{a}Samples reporting more than one positive result in a primary class are counted only once.

(152 samples), and Michigan (145 samples). The distribution of positives among the different drug classes for these individual states is shown in Figs. 5–10, respectively. These figures show that, although alcohol was the most predominant drug among all the six states, there were differences in the predominance of the other drugs. While amphetamines were the second most predominant drug class in California, benzodiazepines were second in Texas and Pennsylvania, and marijuana was second in New York, Florida, and Michigan. Table 4 shows the number of samples received from each state and the distribution of positives among the different drug classes by state.

Urine Sample Analysis

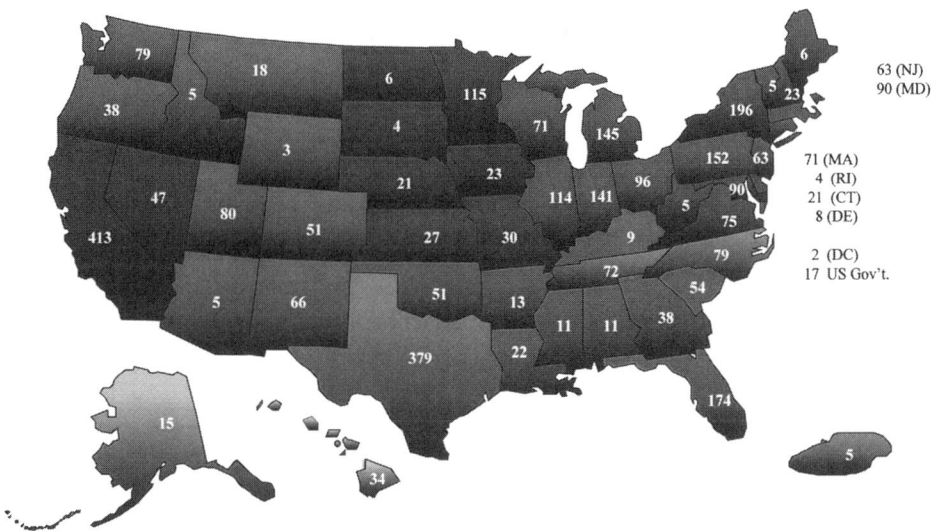

Fig. 4. Number of samples submitted by the different states.

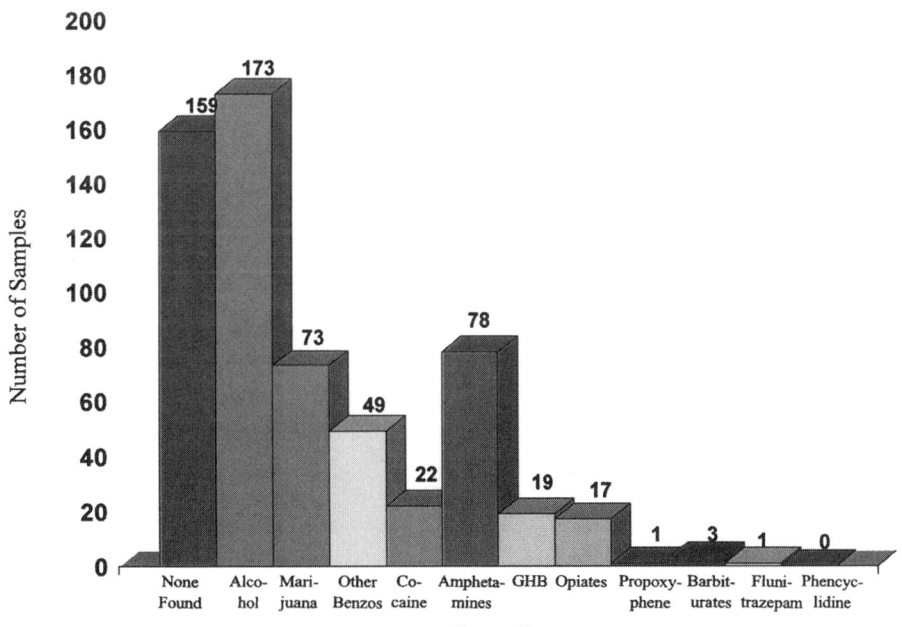

Fig. 5. Distribution of positives confirmed by GC/MS among the 413 samples analyzed from the state of California. Some samples contain more than one substance.

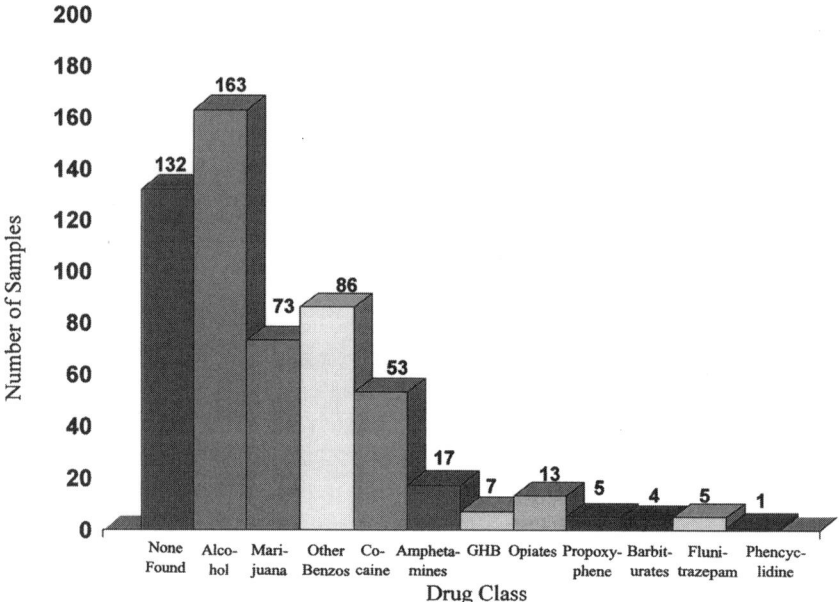

Fig. 6. Distribution of positives confirmed by GC/MS among the 379 samples analyzed from the state of Texas. Some samples contain more than one substance.

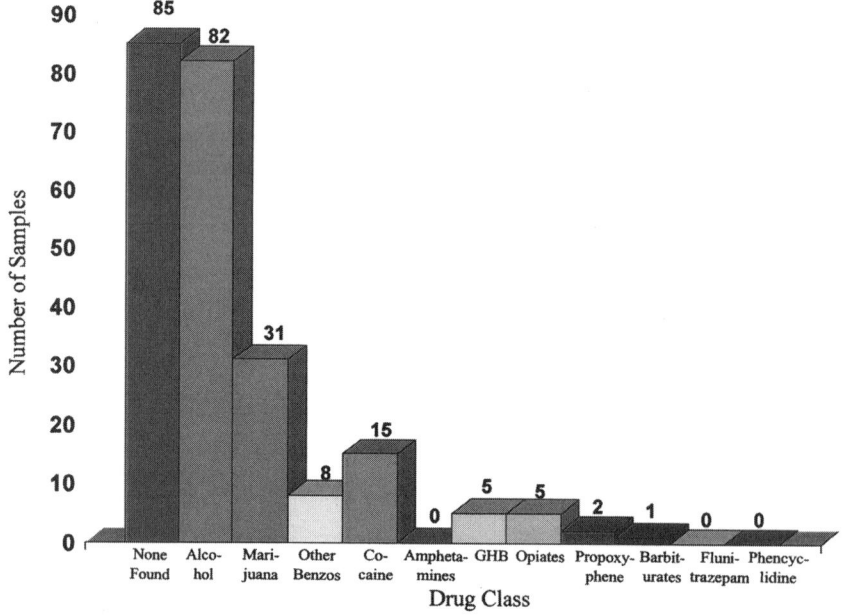

Fig. 7. Distribution of positives confirmed by GC/MS among the 196 samples analyzed from the state of New York. Some samples contain more than one substance.

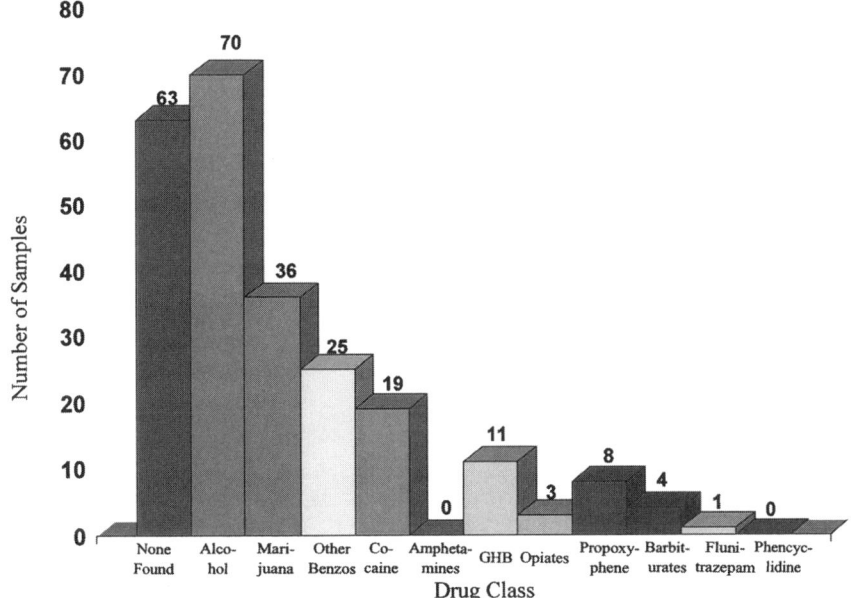

Fig. 8. Distribution of positives confirmed by GC/MS among the 174 samples analyzed from the state of Florida. Some samples contain more than one substance.

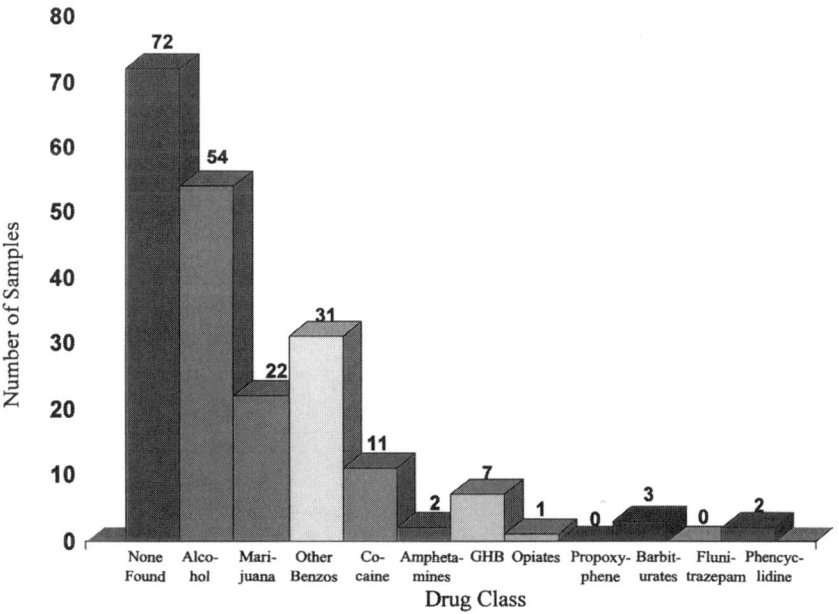

Fig. 9. Distribution of positives confirmed by GC/MS among the 152 samples analyzed from the state of Pennsylvania. Some samples contain more than one substance.

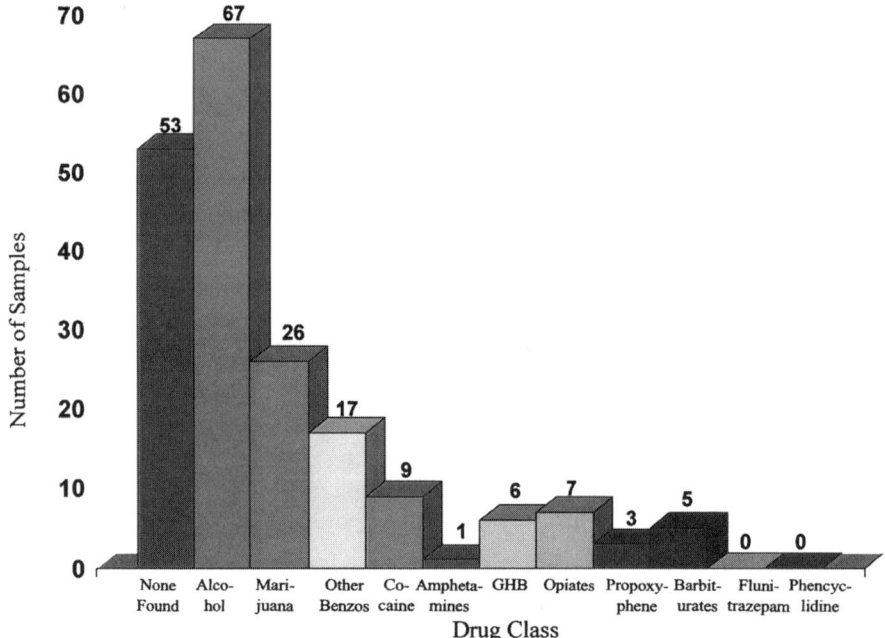

Fig. 10. Distribution of positives confirmed by GC/MS among the 145 samples analyzed from the state of Michigan. Some samples contain more than one substance.

Table 4
Distribution of Positives
Among the Different Drug Classes for Samples Submitted by Each State

State	No. of samples	None found	FN	EtOH	THC	Other benzo-diazepam	AMP	COC	GHB	OPI	PPXY	BARB	PCP	Other drugs
AK	15	5	0	6	5	4	6	2	0	0	0	1	0	0
AL	11	3	0	4	1	7	0	0	0	1	1	0	0	0
AR	13	7	1	3	0	4	0	0	0	0	0	0	0	0
AZ	5	1	0	4	1	0	0	1	0	0	0	0	0	0
CA	413	159	1	173	73	49	78	22	19	17	1	3	0	0
CO	51	18	0	25	7	4	4	5	0	0	0	0	0	0
CT	21	14	0	3	5	3	0	0	0	0	0	0	0	0
DE	8	3	0	4	1	2	0	0	0	0	0	1	0	0
FL	174	63	1	70	36	25	0	19	11	3	8	4	0	0
GA	38	18	0	14	6	3	0	1	1	0	0	1	0	0
HI	34	9	0	9	12	11	10	4	0	2	0	1	0	0
IA	23	13	0	8	3	4	4	0	0	0	0	0	0	0
ID	5	4	0	0	1	0	0	0	0	0	1	0	0	0
IL	114	53	0	43	14	13	4	8	8	2	1	1	0	0
IN	141	44	0	61	40	35	7	11	1	6	3	2	0	0

(*continued*)

Urine Sample Analysis

State	No. of samples	None found	FN	EtOH	THC	Other benzo-diazepam	AMP	COC	GHB	OPI	PPXY	BARB	PCP	Other drugs
KS	27	14	0	10	2	0	0	1	0	2	0	0	0	0
KY	9	2	0	4	2	3	0	0	1	0	0	0	0	0
LA	22	7	0	8	6	9	2	3	3	1	1	0	0	0
MA	71	28	0	29	9	12	1	6	1	6	0	0	0	0
MD	90	33	0	39	18	9	2	9	6	3	2	1	0	0
ME	6	3	0	2	2	2	0	1	0	0	0	0	0	0
MI	145	53	0	67	26	17	1	9	6	7	3	5	0	0
MN	115	35	1	62	21	12	6	14	2	3	0	0	0	0
MO	30	15	0	10	3	2	2	0	1	0	0	1	0	0
MS	11	7	0	3	1	0	0	0	0	0	1	0	0	0
MT	18	8	0	6	2	1	2	0	1	0	1	0	0	0
NC	79	22	0	42	16	14	1	6	0	2	0	0	0	0
ND	6	3	0	2	0	0	0	0	1	1	0	0	0	0
NE	21	6	0	13	4	3	0	1	1	0	1	0	0	0
NH	23	11	0	4	8	2	0	2	1	0	0	1	0	0
NJ	63	30	0	20	12	10	2	9	1	1	0	0	0	0
NM	66	24	0	28	9	12	8	12	0	1	0	1	0	0
NV	47	14	0	22	8	3	12	3	0	0	1	0	0	0
NY	196	85	0	82	31	8	0	15	5	5	2	1	0	0
OH	96	33	1	44	18	12	0	7	3	4	3	3	0	0
OK	51	19	1	20	12	16	10	0	2	0	1	2	0	0
OR	38	14	0	12	10	5	8	1	2	1	1	1	0	0
PA	152	72	0	54	22	31	2	11	7	1	0	3	2	0
RI	4	2	0	2	0	0	0	0	0	0	0	0	0	0
SC	54	23	0	24	10	2	1	4	1	0	2	0	0	0
SD	4	3	0	1	0	0	0	0	0	0	0	0	0	0
TN	72	27	0	24	19	27	2	12	1	0	1	0	0	0
TX	379	132	5	163	73	86	17	53	7	13	5	4	1	0
UT	80	25	0	34	19	14	18	9	2	1	0	0	0	0
VA	75	28	0	32	14	8	0	5	4	2	1	2	0	0
VT	5	3	0	2	0	0	0	0	0	0	0	0	0	0
WA	79	27	0	27	23	12	10	7	1	2	2	1	0	0
WI	71	36	0	27	8	1	0	5	0	0	1	0	0	0
WV	5	2	0	3	0	4	0	1	0	0	0	0	0	0
WY	3	3	0	0	0	0	0	0	0	0	0	0	0	0
DC	2	1	0	1	0	0	0	0	0	0	0	0	0	0
PR	5	4	0	1	0	0	0	1	0	0	0	0	0	0
Other	17	9	0	7	0	1	0	0	0	0	0	0	0	0
Total	3303	1277	11	1358	613	502	220	279	100	87	44	40	3	0

To determine the effect of time lapse from incident to collection on the possibility of detecting drug use, the data for the positive samples were analyzed by time interval. Table 5 shows the number of positive samples detected for each drug class by 12-h segments. It is clear from the data in Table 5 that the majority of positive samples for all drugs were those collected within the first 24 h post-incident. Therefore, it is recommended that for investigation of drug facilitated sexual assault, specimens should be collected as soon as possible

Table 5
Distribution of Positive Samples
Among the Different Drug Classes by Time of Collection

Primary drug class	0–12	13–24	25–36	37–48	49–72	>72	Unknown	Total
Alcohol	775	458	40	39	35	3	6	1356
Amphetamines	45	46	10	11	3	0	1	116
Barbiturates	8	12	6	6	6	0	1	39
Benzo/flunitrazepam	4	7	0	0	0	0	0	11
Cocaine	110	111	16	24	14	2	2	279
GHB	43	37	8	7	5	0	0	100
Marijuana	211	252	49	49	47	2	3	613
Opiates	20	21	2	9	4	0	0	56
Other benzodiazepines	95	130	30	25	20	0	4	304
Phencyclidine	1	2	0	0	0	0	0	3
Propoxyphene	17	19	1	1	4	0	2	44
	1329	1095	162	171	138	7	19	2921

after the incident. This is particularly important for some of the drugs with short half life such as alcohol and GHB.

5. CONCLUSIONS

This study was initiated to determine the prevalence of drug use among alleged drug-facilitated sexual assault victims, with particular interest in the prevalence of flunitrazepam. Urine specimens were collected from a total of 3303 alleged sexual assault victims claiming that the assault was drug-facilitated, and the specimens were analyzed for different drugs of abuse by commonly available immunoassays to identify presumptive positives. Specimens that screened positive were confirmed by GC/MS. For flunitrazepam, however, every specimen was analyzed by a very sensitive GC/MS procedure to assure that, if the drug had been involved in the assault, it would have been detected, even if the specimen was collected as late as 72 h post-ingestion.

The study covered the period from May, 1996, to February, 2000, and a total of 3303 specimens were submitted by law enforcement agencies, rape crisis centers, and emergency rooms treating sexual assault victims. The results of testing showed that 62.3% of the samples were positive for at least one drug, of which 36% were positive for two or more drugs. The drug most frequently found in the submitted specimens was alcohol, followed by marijuana, benzodiazepines, cocaine, amphetamines, and GHB in a descending order. The pattern of prevalence of the different drugs was different from state to state. While amphetamines and GHB were most predominant in California, benzodiazepines and cocaine were most predominant in Texas. The state of Texas also provided the highest number for flunitrazepam positives (almost 50% of all positive flunitrazepam samples in the study). On the other hand, Florida provided the highest number of propoxyphene positives, and Pennsylvania provided two out of the three phencyclidine positives.

Several conclusions could be drawn from careful examination of the data:

1. Alcohol was the most predominant drug found in the specimens analyzed.
2. There was a high rate of multiple drug use not necessarily limited to CNS depressant drugs.
3. There was a relatively high incidence of GHB positives. GHB is a potent tranquilizer with a short half life and, therefore, should be included in any forensic examination of sexual assault cases.
4. Aside from alcohol, there is no one class of drugs that could be considered as being strongly associated with sexual assault.
5. The rate of positives for flunitrazepam was exceptionally low (0.33%). The association of flunitrazepam with alleged sexual assault has been highly exaggerated.
6. A wide range of drugs could be involved in sexual assault cases.
7. Most of the positive samples were found in specimens collected within 24 h postincident. Current technologies, including sensitive immunoassays and GC/MS, allow the detection of most drug classes within this time frame.
8. Sexual assault kits should include a urine collection container, and urine should be collected.
9. It is important to remember that the mere presence of drug(s) in a urine specimen does not necessarily mean that the drug was administered as a part of the alleged sexual assault.

It is unfortunately true that many substances have been (and will be) used in attempted sexual assaults. However, urine samples from alleged sexual assault victims who believed they were given drugs prior to sexual assault were found to contain alcohol and/or prescription medications such as codeine, several benzodiazepines and amphetamines, as well as a number of illegal drugs including marijuana and cocaine.

References

1. Koss, M. P., Dinero, T. E., and Seibel, C. A. (1988) Stranger and acquaintance rape: are there differences in the victim's experience? *Psychol. Women Q* **12,** 1–24.
2. Muehlenhard, C. L. and Linton, M. A. (1987) Date rape and sexual aggression in dating situations: incidence and risk factors. *J. Couns. Psychol.* **34,** 186–196.
3. Anonymous (1997) Gamma hydroxy butyrate use—New York and Texas, 1995–1996. *MMWR* **46,** 281–323.
4. Masters, B. A. (1997) Date rape drugs. *Washington Post*, March 24.
5. Merle, R. (1997) "Special-K" is latest U.S. drug fad. *The Seattle Times*, June 20.

6. Anglin, D., Spears, K. L., and Hutson, H. R. (1997) Flunitrazepam and its involvement in date or acquaintance rape. *Acad. Emer. Med.* **4**, 323–326.
7. Woods, J. H. and Winger, G. (1997) Abuse liability of flunitrazepam. *J. Clin. Psychopharmacol.* **17**, 1–57.
8. ElSohly, M. A., Feng, S., Salamone, S. J., and Wu, R. (1997) A sensitive GC/MS procedure for the analysis of flunitrazepam and its metabolites in urine. *J. Analyt. Toxicol.* **21**, 335–340.
9. Salamone, S. J., Honasoge, S., Brenner, C., McNally, A. J., Passarelli, J., Goc-Szkutnicka, K., et al. (1997) Flunitrazepam excretion patterns using the Abuscreen OnTrak and OnLine immunoassays: comparison with GC/MS. *J. Analyt. Toxicol.* **21**, 341–345.
10. Ferrara, S. D., Tedeschi, L., Frison, G., Castagna, F., Gallimberti, L., Giorgetti, R., et al. (1993) Gamma-hydroxybutyric acid monitoring in plasma and urine by gas chromatography-mass spectrometry. *J. Pharm. Biomed. Anal.* **11**, 483–487.

Index

Alcohol, *see* Sexual assault
Alprazolam,
   electron capture detection, 55, 57
   gas chromatography-mass spectrometry analysis,
      conditions, 58
      extraction, 57, 58
      overview, 55, 57
      performance, 58, 59
   half-life, 53, 54
   high-performance liquid chromatography-mass spectrometry analysis,
      advantages, 59, 60
      chromatography conditions, 60
      extraction, 60
      performance, 60, 63
      tandem mass spectrometry, 60
   immunoassay limitations, 53, 55, 57
   pharmacokinetics, 56, 57
   therapeutic dose, 53-55
   uses, 53, 54
γ–Aminobutyric acid (GABA),
   postmortem production of γ–hydroxybutyric acid, 111
   receptors,
      benzodiazepine binding, 9–11
      γ–hydroxybutyric acid binding, 98
      subtypes, 8
      subunits, 8, 9
   structure, 96
Amphetamines, *see* Sexual assault
Ativan, *see* Lorazepam

B

Barbiturates, *see* Sexual assault,
Benzodiazepines, *see also* specific drugs,
   abuse liability, 11, 12
   chemistry, 2–4
   hair analysis, *see* Hair, benzodiazepine analysis

Benzodiazepines, *see also specific drugs (cont.)*,
   immunoassays, *see* Immunoassay, benzodiazepines
   overview, 1, 17, 77
   pharmacokinetics, 3, 17, 18
   sexual assault studies, *see* Sexual assault
1,4-Butanediol,
   anesthetic activity, 97
   gas chromatography-mass spectrometry analysis, 118, 119
   illicit use history, 104
   metabolism, 107, 108
   pharmacokinetics, 110
   synonyms, 104, 105
   uses, 104
γ–Butyrolactone (GBL),
   analysis,
      extraction,
         liquid-liquid extraction, 116, 117
         solid-phase extraction, 117, 118
      mass spectrometry, 116, 118
      overview, 115, 116
   anesthetic activity, 97
   γ–hydroxybutyric acid equilibrium, 115
   illicit use history, 102–104
   metabolism, 107
   pharmacokinetics, 103, 104, 110
   scheduling, 102
   synonyms, 103
   synthesis, 103
   uses, 103

C

Capillary zone electrophoresis (CZE), midazolam analysis, 65, 66
CEDIA, *see* Immunoassay, benzodiazepines
Cocaine, *see* Sexual assault
CZE, *see* Capillary zone electrophoresis

D

Date-rape drugs, *see* Flunitrazepam; γ–Hydroxybutyric acid; Sexual assault

E

EMIT, *see* Immunoassay, benzodiazepines

F

Flunitrazepam,
 ability to concentrate versus plasma levels, 13
 acute effect, 10, 11
 date-rape,
  analysis of victim urine samples, *see* Sexual assault
  use, 13, 14, 128
 γ–aminobutyric acid receptor binding, 9-11
 gas chromatography-mass spectrometry,
  analyte retention time and sensitivity, 48, 128
  dual derivatization, 47
  enzyme hydrolysis, liquid-liquid extraction, and derivatization, 46
  hair analysis, 47, 48, 90
  hydrolysis and derivatization, 44
  overview, 43, 44
  sensitivity, 46
  solid-phase extraction, 47
  standards, 44–46
 high-performance liquid chromatography assays,
  detection,
   mass spectrometry, 42, 43, 49
   ultraviolet, 42
  extraction,
   immunoaffinity extraction, 41
   liquid-liquid extraction, 38
   solid-phase extraction, 39–41
   reversed-phase chromatography, 41, 42
   standards, 37, 38
 immunoassay systems,
  EMIT, 35
  enzyme-linked immunosorbent assay, 37
  FPIA, 35
  Micro-Plate Enzyme Immunoassay, 36
  OnLine, 36
  OnTrak, 36
  overview, 35
  radioimmunoassay, 36, 37
 manufacturers, 128
 pharmacokinetics,
  absorption, 4, 5
  distribution, 5, 6
  excretion, 8
  half-life versus duration of action, 7
  metabolism, 3, 7, 8, 33, 34
  plasma levels, 6, 12, 13
 recreational use and abuse, 2, 13
 scheduling, 2, 33
 sedative effects versus plasma levels, 12, 13
 smuggling, 127, 128
 uses and popularity, 1, 2, 127

FPIA, *see* Immunoassay, benzodiazepines

G

GABA, *see* γ–Aminobutyric acid
Gas chromatography-mass spectrometry (GC/MS),
 alprazolam analysis,
  conditions, 58
  extraction, 57, 58
  overview, 55, 57
  performance, 58, 59
 1,4-butanediol analysis, 118, 119
 flunitrazepam analysis,
  analyte retention time and sensitivity, 48, 128
  dual derivatization, 47
  enzyme hydrolysis, liquid-liquid extraction, and derivatization, 46
  hair analysis, 47, 48, 90
  hydrolysis and derivatization, 44
  overview, 43, 44
  sensitivity, 46
  solid-phase extraction, 47
  standards, 44–46
 high-performance liquid chromatography-mass spectrometry analysis,
  atmospheric pressure chemical ionization, 64, 65
  electrospray ionization, 65
 γ–hydroxybutyric acid analysis, 116, 118
 lorazepam analysis,
  conditions, 67
  extraction, 66, 67
  overview, 55, 66
  performance, 67
  tandem mass spectrometry, 67
 midazolam analysis,
  conditions, 64
  extraction, 63, 64
  overview, 55
  performance, 64
 sexual assault, Roche program for drug urine analysis,
  amphetamines, 129
  barbiturates, 129
  benzophenones, 130
  cannabinoids, 129
  cocaine, 129
  flunitrazepam, 130, 142
  opiates, 129
 triazolam analysis,
  extraction, conditions, and performance,
   method 1, 70
   method 2, 71
  overview, 55, 68–70

GBL, *see* γ–Butyrolactone
GC/MS, *see* Gas chromatography-mass spectrometry
GH, *see* Growth hormone
GHB, *see* γ–Hydroxybutyric acid

Index

β–Glucuronidase, benzodiazepine immunoassay utilization,
  calculations of hydrolysis, 21, 22
  catalytic efficiency with different drugs, 19
  incubation conditions, 18
  manual versus automated treatment, 19, 20, 28
  optimal reaction conditions, 19
  pH optimum, 19
  rationale, 18, 23, 24
  sensitivity effects of hydrolysis, 23
  units of activity, 20, 21
Growth hormone (GH), γ–hydroxybutyric acid response, 98, 99

H

Hair, benzodiazepine analysis,
  composition and biology of hair, 78
  cosmetic treatment effects, 80
  decontamination procedures, 81, 82
  detection techniques, 84, 86
  drug incorporation mechanisms, 79, 80
  extraction, 84, 85
    hydrolysis conditions by drug, 81, 83
    pulverization, 81
  flunitrazepam gas chromatography-mass spectrometry analysis, 47, 48, 90
  growth of hair, 78, 79
  historical perspective, 78
  levels by drug, 84, 88-90
  quality assurance, 92
  sensitivity, 77, 84, 86
  specimen collection, 81
  types of hair, 79
High-performance liquid chromatography-mass spectrometry (HPLC/MS),
  alprazolam analysis,
    advantages, 59, 60
    chromatography conditions, 60
    extraction, 60
    performance, 60, 63
    tandem mass spectrometry, 60
  flunitrazepam assays,
    detection,
      mass spectrometry, 42, 43, 49
      ultraviolet, 42
    extraction, 38, 39-41
    reversed-phase chromatography, 41, 42
    standards, 37, 38
  triazolam analysis, 69
HPLC/MS, *see* High-performance liquid chromatography-mass spectrometry
γ–Hydroxybutyric acid (GHB),
  addiction and withdrawal, 98, 100, 101
  alcohol combination, 100
  analysis,
    extraction,
      liquid-liquid extraction, 116, 117
      solid-phase extraction, 117, 118
    mass spectrometry, 116, 118
    overview, 115, 116

γ–Hydroxybutyric acid (GHB) *(cont.)*,
  blood concentration versus state of consciousness, 95, 96
  γ-butyrolactone equilibrium, 115
  clinical uses, 101, 102
  elimination, 109, 110
  growth hormone response, 98, 99
  history of use, 95
  illicit use, 98–101
  metabolism, 104-107
  metabolites, *see* 1,4-Butanediol; γ–Butyrolactone
  neurotransmitter effects, 97, 98
  pharmacokinetics, 96, 108–110
  postmortem production,
    blood samples, 112–115
    cerebrospinal fluid samples, 114
    eye fluid samples, 114
    mechanisms, 110–112
    storage effects in samples, 113, 114
    urine samples, 112, 113, 115
  receptors, 98
  scheduling, 102
  sexual assault analysis of urine samples, *see* Sexual assault
  slang names, 99
  structure, 96
  synthesis, 95, 100
  tissue distribution, 108, 109
  toxicity, 100

I

Immunoassay, benzodiazepines,
  COBAS INTEGRA 700 online assay, 29
  commercial products, 18, 25-27
  comparison of assays,
    CEDIA, 25
    EMIT, 25
    FPIA, 25
    OnLine, 25, 26
    SBENZ, 26
    table, 27
  cross-reactivity of metabolites, 23, 24
  cutoff, 22
  flunitrazepam assays, *see* Flunitrazepam
  β-glucuronidase utilization,
    calculations of hydrolysis, 21, 22
    catalytic efficiency with different drugs, 19
    incubation conditions, 18
    manual versus automated treatment, protocols, 28
    uses, 19, 20
    optimal reaction conditions, 19
    pH optimum, 19
    rationale, 18, 23, 24
    sensitivity effects of hydrolysis, 23
    units of activity, 20, 21
  Hitachi 717 online assay, 28
  optimization of automated assays, 29
  sensitivity, 17, 18, 23, 29
  specificity, 24, 25

L

Lorazepam,
- electron capture detection, 55
- enantiomer separation, 67
- gas chromatography-mass spectrometry analysis,
  - conditions, 67
  - extraction, 66, 67
  - overview, 55, 66
  - performance, 67
  - tandem mass spectrometry, 67
- half-life, 53, 54
- immunoassay limitations, 53, 55
- pharmacokinetics, 66
- therapeutic dose, 53, 54
- uses, 53, 54, 66

M

Marijuana, *see* Sexual assault

Midazolam,
- capillary zone electrophoresis analysis, 65, 66
- electron capture detection, 55
- formulations, 63
- gas chromatography-mass spectrometry analysis,
  - conditions, 64
  - extraction, 63, 64
  - overview, 55
  - performance, 64
- half-life, 53, 54
- high-performance liquid chromatography-mass spectrometry analysis,
  - atmospheric pressure chemical ionization, 64, 65
  - electrospray ionization, 65
- immunoassay limitations, 53, 55
- pharmacokinetics, 63
- therapeutic dose, 53, 54
- uses, 53, 54

P

Pharmacokinetics,
- alprazolam, 56, 57
- benzodiazepines, 3, 17, 18
- 1,4-butanediol, 110
- γ-butyrolactone, 103, 104, 110
- flunitrazepam,
  - absorption, 4, 5
  - distribution, 5, 6
  - excretion, 8
  - half-life versus duration of action, 7
  - metabolism, 3, 7, 8, 33, 34
  - plasma levels, 6, 12, 13

Pharmacokinetics *(cont.)*,
- γ-hydroxybutyric acid, 96, 108–110
- lorazepam, 66
- midazolam, 63
- triazolam, 68

R

Rohypnol, *see* Flunitrazepam

S

Sexual assault, Roche program for drug urine analysis,
- distribution of drugs,
  - alcohol, 131, 142, 143
  - benzodiazepines, flunitrazepam, and clonazepam, 131–135
  - geographic distribution of samples, 134, 136–143
  - marijuana, 131
  - multiple-positive samples, 133, 134, 136, 143
  - time of collection effects, 141, 142
- ethanol analysis, 130
- gas chromatography-mass spectrometry,
  - amphetamines, 129
  - barbiturates, 129
  - benzophenones, 130
  - cannabinoids, 129
  - cocaine, 129
  - flunitrazepam, 130, 142
  - opiates, 129
- immunoassays, 129
- specimen,
  - criteria, 131
  - receipt, 128, 129

T

Triazolam,
- electron capture detection, 55
- gas chromatography-mass spectrometry analysis,
  - extraction, conditions, and performance, method 1, 70
  - method 2, 71
  - overview, 55, 68–70
- half-life, 53, 54
- high-performance liquid chromatography-mass spectrometry analysis, 69
- immunoassay limitations, 53, 55, 68
- pharmacokinetics, 68
- therapeutic dose, 53, 54, 68
- uses, 53, 54

V

Versed, *see* Midazolam

RA
1242
.B43
B465

49014